Conducting GCP-compliant
Clinical Research

Conducting GCP-compliant Clinical Research

Wendy Bohaychuk
and
Graham Ball

Good Clinical Research Practices, UK and Canada

JOHN WILEY & SONS

Chichester • New York • Weinheim • Brisbane• Singapore • Toronto

Other Wiley Editorial Offices

John Wiley & Sons, Inc., 605 Third Avenue,
New York, NY 10158-0012, USA

WILEY-VCH Verlag GmbH, Pappelallee 3,
D-69469 Weinheim, Germany

Jacaranda Wiley Ltd, 33 Park Road, Milton,
Queensland 4064, Australia

John Wiley & Sons (Asia) Pte Ltd, Clementi Loop #02-01,
Jin Xing Distripark, Singapore 129809

John Wiley & Sons (Canada) Ltd, 22 Worcester Road,
Rexdale, Ontario M9W 1L1, Canada

Library of Congress Cataloging-in-Publication Data

Bohaychuk, Wendy.
   Conducting GCP-compliant clinical research / by Wendy Bohaychuk
   and Graham Ball.
       p.   cm.
   Includes bibliographical references and index.
   ISBN 0-471-98824-3 (alk. paper)
       1. Clinical trials–Standards.   2. Drugs–Testing–Standards.
   I. Ball, Graham.   II. Title.   III. Title: Conducting GCP compliant
   clinical research.
   R853. C55B64   1999
   615′. 1901–dc21   –dc21
   [615′. 1901]   98-54676
                                                               CIP

British Library Cataloguing in Publication Data

A catalogue record for this book is available from the British Library

ISBN 0 471 98824 3

Typeset in 11/13 Palatino by Acorn Bookwork, Salisbury, Wilts
Printed and bound in Great Britain by Biddles, Guildford, Surrey
This book is printed on acid-free paper responsibly manufactured from sustainable
forestry, in which at least two trees are planted for each one used for paper production

Contents

Abbreviations

ADR	adverse drug reaction
AE	adverse event
CIOMS	Council for International Organizations of Medical Sciences
CRA	clinical research associate
CRF	case report form (case record form)
CRO	contract research organisation
CV	curriculum vitae
DQF	data query form
EMEA	European Medicines Evaluation Agency
FDA	Food and Drug Administration (USA)
GCP	good clinical practice
GLP	good laboratory practice
GMP	good manufacturing practice
IB	investigator brochure
ICH	International Conference on Harmonisation
IRB	Institutional Review Board
NCR	no carbon/copying required
SAE	serious adverse event
SOP	standard operating procedure
WHO	World Health Organization

Subject	patient volunteer or healthy volunteer
Monitor	person who monitors the study. *The title of this individual may differ according to Sponsor and/or CRO preferences and could be the clinical monitor, clinical research associate (CRA), medical director, etc.*

Introduction

The overall aim of this work is to provide a reference book which describes the general framework for conducting GCP-compliant clinical research, particularly pharmaceutical industry clinical research. Hopefully, it is written in simple enough language so that it is readable to those who are new to the business: however, we have also included many examples from our years of practice to sustain the interest of a more experienced group. Pharmaceutical industry personnel (e.g. monitors, data management personnel, statisticians, medical advisers, and study medication or device suppliers from both sponsors and CROs) will find many helpful hints and examples of how the situation can go awry. We also hope the book will be of value to new and experienced personnel at clinical study sites including investigators, research nurses, study site co-ordinators, clinical laboratory staff and pharmacists. Members of ethics committees and IRBs should find this reference book useful to increase their understanding of how clinical research operates from the perspective of the pharmaceutical industry, and auditors and inspectors will especially find the book helpful because of the numerous references to audit findings. There might be interest from an academic perspective as well.

First of all, we should make it clear that in our opinion there is no such thing as a fully GCP-compliant clinical study. It is almost impossible to achieve the ideal proclaimed in the existing guidelines and regulations. However, this does not mean we should not strive for the best standard possible. You must think beyond the 'minimum standard' if you really want to do a good job and ensure the best quality possible. Slavish adherence to guidelines and regulations will not work: you must be convinced of the basic logic, ethics and science behind GCP requirements. Going for the most expedient and cheapest route will not only result in a poorer standard but it may also cost lives.

How much non-compliance should we tolerate? In 1996, we published a book on GCP compliance based on the findings of our audit experience at 226 investigator study sites, involving studies conducted in 20 different countries, and audited by an independent external audit team between 1991 and 1995. GCP compliance was compared for various factors and the data patterns suggested some interesting trends. First, the overall level of GCP compliance was generally poor across all investigator study sites and far below the expectations of guidelines and regulations. (In many areas, the studies were possibly dangerous for study subjects, in our opinion.) Second, there were no important differences in studies with regard to the year in which the study was conducted. Basically, all the new regulatory efforts, particularly in Europe, did not show a positive effect on standards. (However, a survey over a five- to six-year time period is possibly too limited to draw conclusions on this point.) Third, there were no important differences in studies which used a CRO (contract research organisation) compared to those which did not. This appears to be because CROs simply follow the standards of the sponsor responsible for the conduct of the study rather than setting consistent and better standards themselves. Fourth, some slight differences between phases of studies were observed, with better compliance in early phase studies. However, this should not be surprising since a Phase I single-centre study with 20 subjects is much easier to control than a Phase III multicentre multinational study involving several hundred study subjects. Fifth, there were some slight differences between therapeutic areas, but this was probably linked to the standards of the sponsor or CRO managing the studies. Sixth, overall, there were no basic overall differences between levels of GCP compliance in different countries. (However, a later analysis of selected items showed some individual differences between countries: for example, direct access to source documents was achieved 100% of the time at US sites, but not as frequently in other countries.) The only apparent important differences in levels of GCP compliance were between the different sponsors (mostly pharmaceutical companies) managing the studies. The main conclusions reached from analysis of this audit database were that overall standards of GCP compliance greatly needed improvement, and that standards were only as good as the sponsor managing the study regardless of where in the world the study was being conducted. In theory, good research could be conducted anywhere provided it was managed properly.

There is a desperate need to fill the educational gaps in our understanding of GCP. Frankly, we are often appalled at how little those who are doing the job understand their responsibilities. CONDUCTING GCP-COMPLIANT CLINICAL RESEARCH IS A SERIOUS UNDERTAKING. The welfare of current study subjects and future patients is at stake and we must never underestimate that the application of GCP requires continuous vigilance and care. We must get our priorities straight first. Investigators complain that 'all this GCP is ruining real science'. The pharmaceutical industry complains that GCP requirements make drug development more expensive and more time-consuming. Ethics committees and IRBs complain (rightly) that they do not simply exist to take care of the pharmaceutical industry and anyway, who is educating them with regard to the new regulations and guidelines? Perhaps the smallest voice of objection has come from the hundreds of thousands of study participants, those for whom we should be most concerned about achieving the right standards. However, the latter situation is changing and the protests of consumer groups, patient advocates, and those who must pay for our healthcare, are probably most responsible for the emergence of the many new guidelines and regulations in the last 15–20 years. (In the United States, these changes occurred much earlier.) The study subject obviously has the most to lose from non-compliance with GCP and we have tried hard to look at GCP from the point of view of what is best for the study subject throughout this book.

Many complain that GCP is a boring topic. We try to overcome this in training courses by providing as many practical examples as possible. In this book, we have also taken the same approach. At the end of each chapter, there is a 'case study' describing all the serious findings of GCP non-compliance at a particular study site. Further, throughout the book, there are 'anecdotes' describing incidents which might help the reader understand certain points. All of these reports are based on true events, but the reader will understand that we have had to anonymize these as much as possible and must forgive us for a few generalisations. Lists of requirements, which might be tedious if they are not relevant to a particular situation, have been presented in checklists so that they can be skipped in the first reading and referenced at a later point. (These checklists are not exhaustive but they might provide a helpful starting point for preparing standard operating procedures.) We have also included our audit findings throughout the text to emphasize the levels of non-compliance with certain requirements. As independent auditors, we are in a wonderful position to be able to present the negative findings as openly as possible. Obviously, it would be difficult for sponsor and CRO personnel, and site personnel, to publicly criticise their operations. We hope readers will resist the temptation to dismiss negative findings. Criticism is not intended to be anti-industry or anti-research – it is intended to be pro-patients. After all, this is what GCP is all about.

CHAPTER 1
The Current Rules for Conducting Clinical Research

Clinical research must be conducted according to a set of standards which has been formalised in many international guidelines and regulations. The ultimate aim is to protect all research participants and assure that only worthwhile treatments are approved for use for future patients. GCP principles, although quite straightforward, are not easy to implement (section 1.1.).

One could ask why we need a set of rules if the requirements are so obvious – after all, reasonably intelligent people at all levels are managing the research activity and surely all physicians consider protection of patients as their primary objective. Unfortunately, experience has shown that the requirements are much more complex than they appear and there are serious conflicts of interest. Pharmaceuticals companies obviously develop products which will make profits, investigators are paid to conduct clinical research, patients in some types of studies may be paid to participate and even ethics committees operate to make a profit (e.g. some IRBs in the USA). Thus the public has demanded some control and regulations have arisen. A brief summary of existing regulations is presented in this chapter, but we hope otherwise, throughout this book, to appeal to a sense of logic, science and ethics which we can all understand (section 1.2).

To make sure the standards for clinical research are set before studies begin and to check on those standards, many systems and process must be established. These are formally undertaken by pharmaceutical companies and CROs in the form of project planning, SOPs, training, monitoring, data processing, etc. (section 1.3).

Where there are regulations, there are usually systems to check on conformity with those regulations. The procedures of auditing and inspection are the most valid means of checking on compliance as they are required, by definition, to be conducted independently of the clinical study process. Auditors and inspectors are supposed to be unbiased in their review. Auditing is usually undertaken by the organisation conducting the research to check on compliance with their own standards and basically to pre-empt the inspectors. Inspectors are there in the interests of the public: they are supposed to be independent of the researchers and other participants, such as ethics commit-tees (section 1.4 and 1.5).

The ultimate in GCP non-compliance is fraud. Although this is a negative topic, and most of us would like to feel it does not happen, unfortunately there have been some serious cases which have been uncovered and brought to the attention of the public. There are probably many other situations which have never been pursued, but everyone needs to be sensitive to this issue and prevent its occurrence (sections 1.6).

1.1   THE BASIC TENETS OF GCP

The primary reason for the presence of a GCP code of practice is to protect human rights. If this simple principle could be remem-bered at all times throughout the research process, many of the so-called vagaries of GCP could be resolved. Unfortunately, it is not so easy to keep this principle foremost when one is trying to get a job done or if there is a conflict of interest.

Collecting honest and accurate data is a major part of GCP to ensure that data have integrity and valid conclusions may be drawn from those data. Data should be reproducible: that is, if the study were to be conducted in a similar population using the same procedures, the results should be the same. After all, the results of clinical research will be imposed on new patients in the future. To help assure us all of the integrity and reproducibility of research results, the whole process should be transparent and that means that everything must be documented so that an external reviewer can verify that the research was actually conducted as the researchers reported that it was conducted. Many systems and processes must be in place to implement GCP and the documentation must clearly indicate compliance with those systems (Checklist 1.1–1).

Checklist 1.1–1. General Systems and Procedures for Implementation of GCP

The following systems and procedures must be established by clinical researchers to ensure compliance with GCP requirements:

- Planning: studies must be conducted for valid (ethical and scientific) reasons;
- Standard operating procedures: research procedures must be declared in writing so that reviewers can determine the standards which are being applied and so that users have a reference point;
- Qualified personnel: all personnel (sponsor/CRO and study site) must be experienced and qualified to undertake assigned tasks. Documentation of qualifications and training must be evident.
- Ethics committee review and approval: all studies must be independently reviewed by ethics committees/IRBs, to assess the risk for study subjects, before clinical studies begin. Review must continue throughout the study.
- Informed consent: all study subjects must be given the opportunity to personally assess the risk of study participation by being provided with certain information. Their assent to participate must be documented.
- Well-designed study: all studies must have a valid study design documented in a protocol so that it can be fully reviewed by all interested parties. The data collection plans, as described in the CRF, are part of the protocol.
- Monitoring: a primary means of quality control of clinical studies

involves frequent and thorough monitoring by sponsor/CRO personnel;

- Control of study medications/devices: the product being studied must be managed so that study subjects ultimately receive a safe product and full accountability can be documented;
- Integrity of data: data must be honest. Data must be reviewed by site personnel, monitors and data processing personnel.
- Quality assurance: systems for assuring quality and for checking quality must be established and followed at all stages;
- Archives: documentation of research activities must be securely retained to provide evidence of activities.

1.2   THE GENERAL REGULATORY FRAMEWORK FOR GCP

(This section is only intended to provide a fairly general review of the regulatory framework and the interested reader is advised to seek expert advice elsewhere.)

The regulatory framework for compliance with research procedures has essentially developed in the last two decades, except for the US where rules were first established in the 1930s. Most countries in the European Union, other countries in Europe (e.g. Hungary, Poland and Switzerland) and Japan have regulations on GCP. Other countries have regulations controlling clinical studies, but not specifically directed to GCP, although they have guidelines on GCP (e.g. Canada and Australia). In this decade, an attempt has been made to harmonise the requirements in the form of an ICH GCP document which has been adapted as regulation by many countries. Some countries have no guidelines or regulations, but guidance for researchers has been provided by organisations such as CIOMS and WHO.

Many researchers try to distinguish between guidelines and regulations, claiming that it is only necessary to comply strictly with the latter. However, if put to the test in court, guidelines would assume a high status: it is best to take them seriously. Much of medical practice is not regulated, but in cases of negligence for example, the court will review the 'state of the art' as the expected standard, much of which is documented in guidelines. The same is true for GCP.

In the last few years, there has been increasing interest in inspection of GCP compliance. Although this has been a regulatory requirement in the USA for many years, inspectorates have only just started in countries such as Austria, Denmark, France, Finland, Germany, Japan, The Netherlands, Norway and Sweden. There are problems in finding good inspectors, in deciding on the final standards for inspections and in imposing sanctions for non-compliance. An interesting recent development has been the initiation of inspections in Europe by the central regulatory authority, the European Medicines Evaluation Agency (EMEA).

Regulation of compliance with requirements by ethics committees is also developing in some parts of the world (e.g. France and Denmark). To date, the US FDA is the only authority which is actively checking on the activities of IRBs by inspection and licensing.

For non-compliance with regulations, only the USA has imposed serious sanctions to date. The 'blacklist' (list of all investigators who have been found to be non-compliant and were barred from clinical research for FDA submissions) is publicly available through freedom of information rules. The USA has vast experience (thousands of inspections) compared to the handful of inspections in other countries. For example, at the time of writing this book, the UK has only conducted a few voluntary inspections.

The consequence of non-compliance with GCP requirements may be serious for the researcher and the sponsor, but in this book we are most interested in the consequences for the study subjects. We have published findings elsewhere to suggest that there could be many improvements in compliance as the events of non-compliance we observe cause us great concern. Therefore, we have included many examples of non-compliance in this book which arise from our own experience as auditors. We hope they are helpful in sensitising the reader to some serious issues.

1.3   STANDARD OPERATING PROCEDURES

One of the requirements of GCP is that sponsors and any CROs to whom they contract research are required to have written standard operating procedures (SOPs) to describe necessary activities to accomplish various tasks. These SOPs are intended to interpret the guidelines and regulations so that they can be applied to a specific organisation and answer the questions of who, when, where, why and how. They also provide the means of documenting compliance with GCP requirements. To implement and enforce the SOPs, other quality assurance and control procedures will be used – including training, monitoring and auditing – which are described in other chapters.

A SOP is a formal document which describes the procedures that will be followed to accomplish various tasks. The style of the text of the SOP should be clear, concise, brief and specific to the subject of the SOP. A SOP should be written to provide instructions for the completion of certain procedures and therefore must not be ambiguous or confusing. Statements concerning the procedures to be followed should be made categorical by the use of such words as 'must' and 'will' (e.g. 'the following procedure must/will be performed'). The word 'may' is to be used only when the conditions are stated (e.g. 'the investigator may enter a patient into the study without patient consent only in an emergency and when the patient is unconscious'). Some guidelines for the format of SOPs are included in Checklist 1.3–1.

All sponsor/CRO personnel will be issued with copies of the most current SOPs and will be required to undertake clinical studies in accordance with those SOPs. They will be required to sign a SOP compliance statement stating that they will conform with the requirements of the SOP and specifying the SOPs under consideration.

SOPs will be reviewed at least annually (or more frequently, if necessary, because of urgently needed changes) to determine whether new SOPs or revisions to existing SOPs are needed. All superseded versions of SOPs must be available for audit and inspection. Thus, all master copies of superseded SOPs must be retained in the clinical study files. Reference copies of SOPs may be distributed to individuals in other departments within the company, if required for the task being undertaken, and may be distributed to other external individuals (e.g. a CRO, if required for the task being undertaken). Documented permission to distribute SOPs externally must be obtained to protect confidentiality. Individual recipients of SOPs should not photo-copy the SOPs or distribute them to other personnel and person-nel leaving the employ of the sponsor/CRO should immediately return SOPs.

Under exceptional circumstances, waivers from the SOPs may be allowed, when it is known in advance that it will not be possible to comply with the SOP. Waivers from SOPs must be requested in writing, with an explanation, and require written approval. Violation of SOPs (deliberately or through negligence) must be documented, with an explanation, and reported imme-diately to a designated person. Consistent and deliberate non-compliance with the SOPs without written authorisation will lead to disciplinary action.

The important topics which should be addressed in SOPs by sponsors and CROs are listed in Checklist 1.3–2. Clinical facil-ities conducting research on behalf of sponsors/CROs are also adopting written standards more frequently today and suggested topics are in Checklist 1.3–3. Of 84 different sets of sponsor/CRO SOPs which we have reviewed in the last few years, many important topics were not addressed: inspection by regulatory authorities (87% of SOPs did not include this topic); selection and management of clinical laboratories (77%); medication/device final disposition and destruction (74%); training and qualifications of personnel (70%); selection and management of CROs (68% of 44 sponsor SOP sets); detection and management of fraud (59%); financial payments to investi-gators (57%); medication/device packaging and labelling (57%); randomisation procedures (54%); auditing (51%); medication/device requisition, shipment, receipt and management at the study site (48%); investigator contracts (43%); standard operat-ing procedures (39%); investigator brochures (39%); clinical study reports (35%); source data verification procedures (35%); filing/archiving (33%); CRF (including diary card, quality of life assessment form, etc.) design (31%); protocol amendments (31%); study site initiation and closure(26%); ethics committees (26%); informed consent procedures (24%); and reporting of AEs (21%).

Checklist 1.3–1. Suggestions for the Format and Contents of SOPs

Each SOP will provide the following information on the first page:
- Title: the title will comprise one or two lines indicating the subject of the SOP;
- SOP number: each SOP will be numbered sequentially using five digits. The first set of three digits identifies a SOP and the second set of two digits indicates the revision number.
- Issue date: this will be the date on which the SOP will take effect. It will be on or after the date of approval.
- Supersedes: the number and date of the SOP which preceded the current SOP will be indicated;
- Last and next review dates: the last review date will be the date on which the SOP was last reviewed. If the SOP remains unchanged after the review, the details for 'supersedes' will not change. The next review date will be the next scheduled date on which the SOP is planned to be reviewed.
- Approved by: the SOPs will be approved, with the dated signatures of at least one senior manager and senior individual in the department to whom the SOP applies. The approvals confirm that the SOPs adequately describe the procedures developed and used by the sponsor/CRO.

Each SOP will include the following sections in the text:
- Table of contents: the table of contents will include a list of items included in the SOP, with page numbers;
- Introduction: the introduction should briefly describe the rationale and scope of the SOP;
- Contents: the contents of the SOP will follow the order noted in the table of contents and, in general, will follow the order in which procedures occur;
- Appendices to the SOP will be numbered and listed in the order in which they are addressed in the SOP. Appendices will be designated by Roman numerals (e.g. Appendix I) and placed at the end of the SOP, with each page numbered.

Checklist 1.3–2. Topics for SOPs for Sponsors/CROs

Sponsors/CROs should address the following topics in SOPs:

- General topics: general quality assurance and quality control procedures; clinical development plans; clinical study plans; clinical study tracking; clinical research personnel qualifications; clinical audits; regulatory authority inspections; fraud;
- Ethics: initial and continuing review by ethics committees/IRBs; membership; working procedures; informed consent; consent forms and information sheets; exceptions to normal informed consent procedures;
- Study setup: investigator brochures; protocols; protocol amendments; CRFs; submissions to regulatory authorities; selection visits; Phase I facilities; agreements (e.g. responsibilities, financial, confidentiality, insurance/indemnity agreements); selection of CROs; selection of clinical laboratories; initiation visits; personnel; startup meetings;
- Monitoring and initial data review: monitoring visits; source data verification; CRF review; CRF tracking; data query; database development, review and lock; data conventions; study subject classification; statistical review;
- Management of study medications/devices and clinical laboratory samples: request for study medications/devices; labelling and packaging; shipment; receipt; control at study sites; dispensing; inventory; compliance with use of study medication/device; final disposition; final reconciliation; recall; reallocation; randomisation procedures; clinical laboratory samples;
- Safety event reporting: definitions; recording and reporting AEs; reporting safety information externally.
- Closing the study: closure visits; clinical study reports; premature termination or suspension; archiving.

Checklist 1.3–3. Topics for SOPs for Investigators

The following topics are suggestions for inclusion in study site SOPs:
- General topics: general quality assurance and quality control procedures; clinical research personnel qualifications; clinical audits; regulatory authority inspections; fraud;
- Ethics: initial and continuing review by ethics committees/IRBs; membership; working procedures; informed consent; consent forms and information sheets; exceptions to normal informed consent procedures;

- Study setup: review of investigator brochures, protocols, protocol amendments, CRFs; agreements (e.g. responsibilities, financial, confidentiality, insurance/indemnity agreements);
- Monitoring and initial data review: monitoring visits; source data verification; data query;
- Management of study medications/devices and clinical laboratory samples: shipment; receipt; control at study sites; dispensing; inventory; compliance with use of study medication/device; final disposition; final reconciliation; randomisation procedures; clinical laboratory samples;
- Safety event reporting: definitions; recording and reporting AEs; recording and reporting AEs to ethics committees;
- Closing the study: review of clinical study reports; premature termination or suspension; archiving.

1.4   CLINICAL RESEARCH AUDITING

Auditing is a means of quality assurance which must be undertaken to assess the quality of the research process and may be conducted at any time during a clinical study to ensure continued compliance with GCP. Almost all aspects of GCP could be audited (Checklist 1.4–1).

Auditing, by definition, must be undertaken by independent personnel who may be employed by the organisation for whom the audits are being conducted (internal auditors) or may be outside the organisation (external auditors). Auditing may be conducted during the study (in-process) which might allow time to correct deficiencies or it may be conducted after studies (post-process) when the findings will be helpful for future studies but may not be useful for the study audited.

An audit plan should be prepared by the sponsor/CRO at least annually and should provide details of the studies subject to audit, allowing sufficient time and resources for 'for cause' or unforseen audits. Selection of the specific studies and investigator sites for audit will be based on criteria such as: studies considered pivotal to regulatory approval and likely to attract the attention of inspection by competent authorities such as the 'adequate and well controlled' studies and studies designed to determine dose will be audited; each monitor will be exposed to an audit each year and investigators who have little or no training in clinical research or who are in need of such training will be selected for audit; study sites in a multicentre study considered to be of primary importance in the audit plan will be those with the highest enrolment; if the study is multinational, a site in each country will be selected for audit; and specific sites depend on factors such as number of patients, number of withdrawals, number of AEs and protocol violations. Other sites will be selected for audit if there is considered to be a problem that could be resolved by audit.

The auditors will notify the clinical research department of impending audits and request establishment of an acceptable time and date. The advance warning time will depend on the type of audit to be undertaken. For site audits, due consideration will be given to the fact that study site personnel need sufficient warning to assemble required documents. The sponsor/CRO will be responsible for ensuring that all relevant staff and documents for each audit will be freely available at the time of the audit (Checklist 1.4–2).

There are several variations for the auditing process, but often audits will be conducted using detailed audit checklists, prepared in advance of the audit by the audit team. (The monitor and other clinical research personnel may have access to the checklists in advance to learn which items attract the attention of auditors.) The audit findings will be documented in a formal audit report that will detail the conduct of the audit and summarise the findings and recommendations. Audit reports should never be issued to investigator site personnel, ethics committees, any other persons external to the company, or personnel within other departments within the company, except with written permission. However, the investigator should be provided with a short summary of the findings and details of any necessary action.

The sponsor/CRO personnel who have been subjected to an audit should prepare a written report addressing each of the auditor's recommendations within a predetermined time period (e.g. two months) after receipt of the initial audit report. (Sometimes the investigator site personnel may be asked to respond to audit findings.) Following receipt of the audit report and discussion of its contents within the clinical research department, the recommendations made will be implemented, where possible, for the current study or taken into account for future studies.

An audit certificate will be issued with audit reports at the completion of each audit. The audit certificate is a statement that an audit has taken place and is not an indication that the study meets the requirements of a regulatory (or competent) authority. Audit certificates are the only part of an audit report that may be disclosed externally, and investigators should expect to find a copy of the audit certificate in the study file.

Checklist 1.4–1. Types of Audits which may be Undertaken to Assess GCP Compliance

The following documents, activities or systems may be subject to audit:

- SOPs – to ensure that the SOPs require compliance with all the appropriate standards of GCP;
- Protocol, amendments and CRFs – to ensure that all the essential items required for the proper conduct of the study are included, and that data required by the protocol are reflected in the design of the CRFs.
- Investigator brochures – to ensure that it contains the appropriate information, that it is up to date and has been approved by the appropriate authorities;
- Qualifications and commitment of sponsor/CRO personnel– to determine that personnel have appropriate experience and training and that they have been instructed in the SOPs, the therapeutic area and GCP. The sponsor/CRO is expected to provide evidence (e.g. current workload, assignment to other studies for other companies, SOP policies) that the monitor has sufficient time to properly monitor their assigned study sites.
- Qualifications of investigators (and other site personnel) – to determine whether the investigator is medically qualified, has experience in the therapeutic area and has conducted clinical research previously.
- Investigator agreements – to verify that the requirements of GCP are appropriately stated. The protocol and agreements covering the conduct of the study, confidentiality, indemnity, insurance and finances will be audited.

- Regulatory reviews/approvals – to ensure that the correct documentation was compiled;
- Ethics: – to determine the compliance of ethics committees/IRBs with membership requirements, and to assess the documents submitted to and reviewed by the committee and the content of the committees' working procedures. The content of all information sheets and consent forms will be audited to ensure that the subject is provided with sufficient information and that the consent procedure is appropriately documented.
- Management of study medication/device: The documentation of the methods of transport and management of the study medications/devices from the manufacturer to the study sites may be reviewed. Storage, dispensing, maintenance of security of randomisation schedules, measures of patient compliance and the final accounting of study medications/devices will be audited at the sponsor/CRO and investigator sites. If contracted facilities are used for any aspect of the management of study medications/devices, these may also be subject to audit.
- Monitoring: each monitor may be exposed to an audit at the beginning of subject enrolment (after four or five subjects have been enrolled) and after the study site has been closed. Monitor reports will be audited to determine that: investigators selected for audit have sufficient staff, study subjects and space to conduct the study; documentation of a retrospective analysis of the study site's patient population to support the projected enrolment of subjects. Monitor reports, telephone contact reports and correspondence describing the procedures for initiating study sites and minutes of investigators' meetings will be reviewed to verify that the selected investigators and her/his staff are properly briefed prior to commencing patient enrolment. Monitor reports and telephone contact reports and correspondence which document monitoring visits during patient enrolment will be assessed for content and frequency of monitoring visits.
- Investigator sites: investigator files may be audited to ensure that they contain all the appropriate documents. The auditors will check that source documents exist for all study subjects and that the study subject records clearly indicate participation in the study. Data recorded in the CRFs of a sample of the study subjects will be compared with the source documents to ensure that source document verification has been adequately conducted by the

monitor. Compliance with the protocol will be determined. All data in CRFs will be verified against the source documents. Methods of correcting data at the investigator site and after the CRFs are retrieved by the sponsor/CRO will be reviewed.

- Clinical laboratories – to determine the adequacy of quality control procedures, validity of reference ranges, and the means of collecting and transporting the blood and other samples;
- AE reporting – to assess the methods of reporting AEs and the reporting of SAEs to the regulatory authorities, investigators and ethics committees/IRBs. During source document verification at study sites, source records will be reviewed to ensure that all AEs reported in the patient records were included in the CRF and vice versa.
- Data display: an audit of the data listings and data display tables compared with data recorded in the CRFs may be conducted. The timeliness of data flow will be assessed.
- Final clinical study reports –to verify consistency of the report with the objectives of the protocol, to ensure that all essential items are included in the report and that text data match data listings and analyses.
- Archives – to ensure that all documents are securely archived.

Checklist 1.4–2. Activities During Investigator Site Audits

The following activities will occur during investigator site audits:*
- The auditors will first conduct an audit of all in-house (on sponsor/ CRO premises) documentation. The auditors will notify the monitor of when this will occur and which documents need to be available.
- The monitor (usually) and/or the auditors will prepare a letter of notification which will be sent to study site personnel, confirming the date and time, agenda, and a list of the items to be accessible to the auditor;
- Sites for audit will be chosen by the auditors in consultation with clinical research personnel;
- Prior to the audit, the sponsor/CRO will provide the auditors with photocopies of CRFs selected by the auditors. The auditors will also inform the monitor of all other documents which must be available

* These procedures may vary slightly between companies.

and of any specific personnel with whom it will be necessary to meet.

- Investigators, other key site personnel, and monitors, will be required to be available at each site audit;
- For audits in countries in which the auditors may not be proficient in the local language, the sponsor/CRO must ensure that personnel are available for the duration of the audit to assist in the translation of documents;
- At the beginning of the audit visit, the auditors will explain the purpose and procedures of the audit to the relevant personnel (e.g. the sponsor/CRO staff/investigators/laboratory staff, etc.) prior to commencing the audit;
- The auditors will prepare a letter indicating that they have had access to confidential documents and that an audit has been conducted. A copy of this letter will be placed in the study site files.
- At the conclusion of each audit visit, the auditors will verbally inform the sponsor/CRO staff, investigators, and laboratory staff, as appropriate, of the main findings.
- The monitor will send a follow-up letter to the site personnel thanking them for their time and explaining some of the major findings. Study site personnel should be informed that they will not receive a full copy of the confidential audit report. The monitor is responsible for following up on all outstanding issues at the study site.

1.5   REGULATORY INSPECTIONS

Regulatory authority inspections are conducted to ensure validity of the data and protection of study subjects, and to compare the practices and procedures of the investigator and the sponsor/CRO with the commitment made in the application for marketing.

Regulatory authority inspectors will usually provide advance notification of pending inspections, normally at least one week in advance. When notification for a regulatory authority inspection is received by any personnel, the designated responsible person must be informed immediately. Investigators must be instructed by study monitors that if notification is sent directly to the investigator, the sponsor/CRO must be informed immediately. If the sponsor/CRO is not invited or allowed to participate in the inspection, the investigator must inform the sponsor/CRO immediately of the results of the inspection and the necessary corrective action. If a report is issued by the inspector at the investigator site, the sponsor/CRO must be provided with a copy of the report. It may be necessary for a monitoring visit or audit visit to be undertaken immediately prior to the planned inspection: this will be particularly important to ensure that all appropriate records are available at the study site.

If the inspection allows participation of the sponsor/CRO personnel, an individual will be appointed to act as the 'escort' for an inspection and to be responsible for ensuring that the following items are in place prior to the inspection: all correspondence with regard to the inspection; establishment of the scope of the inspection and confirmation with the inspector; organisation of times and dates, places, and any necessary travel; assembly of required documentation (and only required documentation); instructions to investigators for conduct during inspections; and organisation of personnel who should also be available during the inspection. In particular, a translator may be required.

In principle, all information relevant to the study should be available for inspectors. In practice, it may not be appropriate to provide some items. The inspector should not routinely be provided with confidential items (e.g. personnel records detailing salary review, sales data, etc). In particular, inspectors should not be provided with internal or external audit reports (Checklist 1.5–1).

If an inspection report is received, the nominated sponsor/ CRO individual should ensure that the report is distributed appropriately. A record must be kept of all recipients of the inspection reports and the original inspection report should be filed in a secure confidential location separate from the clinical study file. If follow-up action is requested by the inspector, the proposed action must be discussed and a sponsor/CRO individual will be assigned to be responsible for any necessary follow-up. Any follow-up activities undertaken must be documented. If a regulatory warning letter has been issued, this must be addressed by a designated sponsor/CRO individual.

Checklist 1.5–1. Conduct During Regulatory Inspections of Study Sites

During a regulatory inspection of a study site, the appointed 'escort' (usually sponsor/CRO personnel) will be responsible for ensuring that all the following activities are handled:

- Meet the inspectors and escort them on the premises on the day of the inspection. At both the sponsor/CRO and study site inspections, the inspectors should not be given free access to personal work areas (e.g. private offices, desks).
- Ask to see the credentials of all inspectors;
- Establish a schedule with the inspector (e.g. interview times, refreshment breaks, lunch, etc.);
- Record minutes of all inspection activities. All significant events and discussions should be recorded in the minutes.
- If relevant, the inspector should be made aware of safety and health policies (e.g. no smoking areas);
- Assist the inspector in retrieving documents during the inspection. It may also be necessary to provide or organise administrative assistance (e.g. telephone, mail, fax, etc.).
- Keep a record of all items photocopied. Ensure that confidentiality is respected (e.g. documents with patient names should not be photocopied unless the names are removed).
- For the 'exit interview', ensure that all appropriate personnel are invited and are present at the meeting.

1.6 FRAUD. THE ULTIMATE NON-COMPLIANCE IN GCP

The ultimate in GCP non-compliance is fraud, which may be broadly defined as a deliberate act of altering, omitting or manufacturing data. It is often undertaken to change eligibility or evaluability criteria so that patients can be recruited to, and remain in, studies. Sometimes, whole patients are invented!

Suspected fraud must be handled with confidentiality, accuracy and objectivity. During the course of monitoring activities, clinical research personnel may detect situations which indicate that there is wilful misrepresentation of the study data (Checklist 1.6–1). All studies will have errors; however, numerous errors or specific patterns of errors may be signs for suspicion. It must always be considered that some events could occur by chance and may not be indicators of fraud. Additionally, some events could occur because of poor monitoring procedures. The situation must be managed carefully as it may be as damaging to wrongfully accuse an individual of wrong-doing as it is to accept data which have not been honestly collected.

... A study which was under suspicion of being fraudulent by the sponsor, was assessed not to be so by the auditors. Nevertheless, the study was not accepted by the French subsidiary for submission to the authorities. To us, this was a case in which a bad name was attached to the study and thus a hint of suspicion resulted in the rejection of some data.

... An investigator in The Netherlands told a story of how he had been involved in uncovering some evidence to convict a fraudulent investigator. Over time, this story was twisted so that eventually he himself was accused of fraud.

A report of suspected fraud should first be discussed with the designated sponsor/CRO personnel. If fraudulent activity is suspected, this should not be recorded in the monitor report or any other documents which form part of the clinical study file which is available for inspection. A separate report, clearly marked confidential, must be prepared. If suspicions are confirmed, a for-cause audit will be initiated. If suspicions are unconfirmed, the situation will be reviewed again in a specified time period (e.g. two months). If an investigation indicates, beyond reasonable doubt, that fraudulent data have been submitted, the sponsor/CRO will be responsible for any reporting to regulatory authorities or other disciplinary bodies.

Checklist 1.6–1. Possible Indications of Fraud

The following events or situations may be possible indicators of fraudulent activity at study sites:
• Lack of substantiation of CRF entries in source documents;
• Absence of source documents or source data;

- Numerous discrepancies between CRFs and source documents;
- Rapid recruitment relative to other centres;
- Lack of expected variation in parameters (e.g. blood pressure, laboratory data, start of dosing or other procedures, sampling times);
- One style of handwriting, other handwriting idiosyncrasies and one pen for several subjects over a long time period;
- One style of completion of forms required to be filled in by different study subjects;
- Inaccurate and inconsistent dates, dates on holidays and weekends, several subjects all starting on the same day, inconsistencies with appointment books;
- No consent forms or suspicious signatures on consent forms;
- Discrepancies in use of study medications/devices (more than was shipped, more than was returned, differences between dispensing records and diary cards, differences between diary cards and CRFs);
- Complete absence of AEs or unusual patterns of AEs;
- 'Perfect' compliance;
- Investigator elusiveness, evasiveness.

CASE STUDY ONE

A Single-centre Double-blind Comparative Study of Drug X in the Treatment of X in Approximately 50 Children (Canada)

Many things went wrong in this study which was still recruiting children at the time of the audit. The first serious finding was that the sponsor was conducting this study without a comprehensive set of SOPs. Many of the deficiencies noted in this study occur in other studies even when SOPs are present, but the chances of eliminating a few of the problems are greater when written operating procedures are available. Would you like your children to go into a study with these standards?

Summary of Major Deficiencies

Standard Operating Procedures: The sponsor did not have any standard operating procedures to cover clinical research activities during the time of the study.

Ethics Committee Review: There was no documentation to indicate that the final study protocol had been approved by the local ethics committees and there was no documentation to indicate that the study had been approved by an ethics committee prior to the first study subject providing consent for the study. The ethics committee approval letters did not refer to the current study in adequate detail (e.g. by exact title, protocol number, protocol version, protocol date). (Approval was sought from one other committee in the same city: the approval letter referred to a study with a different disease using the same investigational drug.)

The documentation in the study file did not indicate exactly which items were reviewed and/or approved by the ethics committee. Several important items were apparently not considered (e.g. consent procedures, confidentiality protection, risks to subjects, compensation or treatment for injury, CRFs, investigator brochure, number of subjects to be studied and means of recruitment and justification of sample size.) There was no evidence of any on-going review by the ethics committee. In particular, details of all protocol amendments and all SAEs were apparently not submitted to the ethics committee. The ethics committee membership list did not provide sufficient details concerning the members. One of the investigators was listed as the chairperson of the ethics committee: there was no indication of whether or not the chairperson abstained from voting for this particular study. (The approval letter did not indicate which members were present at the meeting.)

Informed Consent Procedures: The first study subject signed a consent form before ethics committee approval. For many subjects, the consent signatures predated the final protocol. There was no explanation in the study files as to why consent was obtained so early. The consent forms did not provide space for signatures or dates of investigators. Physicians (some of whom were research fellows) who were providing information to obtain consent were not formally delegated as investigators.

The consent form and information sheet were not prepared in a language which was technically appropriate for the study subjects. They were also missing many important items. In particular, the following significant items were missing: a clear indication that the sponsor would be reviewing personal medical records; a full description of the procedures to be followed in the study; a clear indication of the required duration of participation in the study; a clear indication of the risks, discomforts, side effects and inconveniences; compensation for injury; and a clear description of measures to be taken in the event of AEs or therapeutic failure.

Protocol: The protocol did not indicate whether or not it was a final version. The sponsor did not have a copy of the protocol signature page indicating approval. The protocol approval page in the investigator files postdated the entry of several subjects to the study.

The protocol did not contain sufficient detail. Among the significant items which were missing from the protocol were: a clear indication of the number of study sites to be involved and the planned recruitment among the study sites; full identification of the sponsor, monitor and investigators; a consistent description of the required duration of participation of each study subject; full details of the evaluability criteria; full details of the management of the study medication; a clear description of AEs and requirements for recording and reporting; a clear indication that direct access to source documents would be required; and a complete description of responsibilities and procedures for data handling and statistical analysis.

The protocol amendment system was inadequate. Six protocol 'modifications' were provided with the protocol for audit. There was no indication whether or not this was the complete set and amendments were not numbered or dated.

CRF Design: The CRF was deficient in the extent and style of recording information. For several parameters, the CRF did not capture data exactly as required by the protocol and the protocol did not provide sufficient detail for design of the CRF. In some cases, there were discrepancies between requirements of the protocol and requirements of the CRF.

Setting Up the Study: An investigator brochure was apparently not in place from the beginning of the study. The investigator brochure was missing several important items with regard to management of the study medication (e.g. summary of possible medication interactions, summary of contraindications and precautions, instructions with regard to management of the study medication such as storage, preparation, dispensing, management of accidental exposure, and management of overdose).

The sponsor files did not clearly provide information concerning all relevant sponsor personnel from the beginning of the study. (A CV was only available for one monitor although apparently at least four were involved in the study.) The sponsor files did not clearly indicate that all responsible sponsor personnel were appropriately trained.

The documentation of the qualifications of the declared investigators did not indicate usual responsibilities (e.g. teaching, clinic, research) and other clinical research commitments. Five other physicians who were undertaking investigator responsibilities for this study were not formally designated as investigators and had not signed the protocol.

Several investigator responsibilities were not specified in the protocol or in other separate contracts (e.g. requirements to review preclinical information, allow direct verification of CRFs against source documents, report SAEs immediately, review and sign the final clinical report, maintain a confidential record to allow unambiguous identification of each study subject, maintain all records for a specified time period, allow independent audit, and work according to GCP (specifically defined or referenced). The sponsor did not have a signed copy of the protocol and did not have written agreement from all investigators to conduct the study in accordance with the protocol.

There was no evidence of a formal site assessment before placement of the study at this particular site. Further, there was no evidence of a formal site initiation. Documentation of 'pretrial' activities postdated the date of first subject consent.

Monitoring: There were no formal monitoring reports for one year after the first subject provided consent. Fulfilment of several important monitoring responsibilities was not described in the monitor reports (e.g. any direct contact with the investigators, review of study medication, review of clinical laboratory documentation, review of samples collected for analyses).

Control of Clinical Study Medication: The storage of the study medication at the sponsor site was inadequate. Bottles of tablets were stored on the floor in an office. Returned tablets were also stored on the floor and had not been checked at the time of the audit (at least two years after the start of the study). There was no temperature control in the office. At the study site, the storage conditions of the medication were not specified. The pharmacist was not able to locate a thermometer or temperature recording or controlling device in the pharmacy of the hospital.

The shipment note and acknowledgement of receipt note did not contain sufficient detail (e.g. method of shipment, handling instructions, storage instructions and expiry dates). Information in the acknowledgement of receipt note indicated a lack of control of shipment and receipt of study medication. Some of the confusing items were: several dates of receipt signatures were two to six days after shipment and there was no explanation for this interval; one receipt form was not dated; several shipments included supplies for compassionate use and it was difficult to determine exactly what was supplied for the study; several different signatures on the forms were illegible; and the receipt date and signature page did not always agree, causing confusion about when the supplies were actually received. There was no indication of control (shipment, receipt, labelling, dispensing, reconciliation) of the comparator medication.

There was some confusion as to whether the investigational drug was dispensed only to study subjects as the shipment notes included supplies for at least one other study. Several discrepancies in accountability of the study medication were not adequately explained. When medication was returned by study subjects, the tablets were placed in bulk containers at the study site so that it was not possible for the sponsor to check the returns of individual study subjects.

Emergency randomisation code envelopes were not secure. (Regular stationary envelopes were used which could have been easily opened and were not lightproof.)

Filing/Archiving: At both sponsor and investigator premises, records were not reasonably secure from threat of theft, fire and water damage. At the sponsor premises, several documents which should have been in secure archives were still in working files. Several documents were missing from both sponsor and investigator files.

Source Data: The source documents did not clearly indicate participation in the study. Visit dates and exposure to the study medication, including changes in dosing, were not consistently reported in the source documents. There was no clear evidence that primary care physicians had been notified of study participation. It appeared that some subjects were randomised to treatment before all baseline assessments had been recorded.

AEs reported in the CRF were not consistently supported in the source documents. Assessment (for clinical significance) of out-of-range laboratory values was not standardised. (This resulted in several data queries for out-of-range values.)

Some documents retained by the sponsor identified subjects by their full name. Changes to data were not always initialled and dated. Data changes were not authorised by investigators. Some data query clarifications were made by the study site data co-ordinator and some of these related to AE data. CRF retrieval by the sponsor and issue of data queries was not prompt. Two-year old data were not yet computerised.

CHAPTER 2
Setting Up Clinical Studies

The sponsor has a duty to place a study safely. That is, the sponsor (or the delegated CRO) must assess and choose a site where study subjects will not be harmed. Some companies report that they have little choice in this process because the marketing department has already selected the investigators (often those most likely to influence use of the medications/devices), or because there are too few patients or investigators in a particular therapeutic area, or because they have been approached by keen investigators. None of these factors is as important as compliance with the basic GCP principle which requires the sponsor/CRO to assess, select and choose safe settings for research. It is not an easy process.

Setting up clinical studies is a lengthy process as there are many documents to prepare (e.g. protocols, CRFs, investigator brochures), study facilities to be assessed (e.g. study sites, CROs, clinical laboratories, Phase I units), regulatory review to be considered, and negotiations and agreements with study sites (e.g. contracts, finances, confidentiality, indemnity, insurance) to be undertaken (sections 2.1– 2.9).

In addition, as will be dealt with in separate chapters, ethical aspects of the study must be considered (e.g. ethics committee/

IRB review and informed consent requirements) and study medications/devices to be organised (e.g. requisition, packaging, labelling and shipment). The latter, in particular, can be demanding if the study is a double-blind comparative study as it is not easy to prepare matching formulations and this is often a rate-limiting step.

The intensity of these activities is reflected in the list of SOP topics held by sponsors and CROs. There are probably more SOPs dealing with pre-study requirements than any other topics. It is no wonder that compliance with these requirements is time-consuming and may take several months. In fact, it could easily take more than a year to set up a multicentre, multinational double-blind study properly. Even a Phase I study, which is normally single-centre, involving fewer study subjects and less complicated medication/device preparation, may take several weeks or months to organise.

Finally, before any study subjects can be treated, there must be an initiation process at all study facilities. Normally, this entails the monitor visiting the study sites to confirm that all prerequisites are still being met (section 2.10).

2.1   PROTOCOLS

The protocol, with the accompanying relevant CRF, is the key document governing a clinical study. It is the primary document for formally describing how a clinical study will be conducted and how the data will be evaluated and it must include all the information that an investigator should know in order to properly select subjects, collect safety and efficacy data and prescribe the correct study medication/device.

Protocols must be prepared in accordance with a specified and standardised format which is described in guidelines and regulations. The reader is particularly advised to refer to the relevant ICH document. The sponsor/CRO must have a good SOP in place to comply with the requirements. Summaries of protocols and other documents 'explaining' the protocol should never substitute for the authorised protocol. These other documents may be useful, but they do not usually go through the same rigorous preparation and review process as the protocol, and as a result they may conflict with the protocol. The protocol is also likely to be the only document formally reviewed externally (e.g. by the ethics committee/ IRB and the regulatory authority).

The CRF is part of the protocol, but unfortunately, the CRF does not accompany the protocol for distribution at more than 50% of study sites in our auditing experience. This occurs because the protocol is usually prepared first and CRFs are prepared some weeks or months later. External reviewers (e.g. ethics committees/IRBs and regulators) rarely see or rarely request CRFs at the time the protocol is assessed, and usually never see this document throughout the study. We think this is a serious deficiency as the CRF provides much detail about the data collection – we advise investigators not to sign protocols until they have also reviewed the final CRF! Only when they review the CRF will they fully appreciate the work involved in data collection.

In pharmaceutical industry research, protocols are often prepared, at least initially, by the sponsor or the delegated CRO. Investigator input is obviously necessary, but it is highly unlikely that a protocol will be prepared solely by an investigator. There are good reasons for this: protocols must comply with regulatory requirements about which investigators are probably not sufficiently knowledgeable; protocols must fit into overall product development plans as it is unethical to conduct studies without good rationale (and it is not good business either); protocols must be standardised across multicentre studies so that it might not be possible to consider individual investigator preferences; and data collection, as described in the protocol, must be in accordance with the capabilities of the data processing group, which is usually handled by the sponsor or CRO. The protocol must be reviewed and approved internally by the sponsor/CRO before being released to the investigators, ethics committees or other external reviewers. Internal (sponsor/CRO) signatures (especially the medical expert and the biostatistician) must be indicated on the protocol signature page in the final protocol designated for external distribution. (In our audit database, 57% of protocols at 226 study sites were not apparently reviewed by a biostatistician.) If a CRO is involved in the study, a representative of the CRO must sign the signature page

– all responsible parties should sign this important document to indicate their review and agreements to comply with the requirements.

Usually, protocols are approved by both the sponsor and the investigator before release to other external reviewers. Therefore, after internal approval and release, all designated investigators, at each study site, must also sign the protocol on the protocol signature page. (Investigators include all physicians who will be undertaking investigator responsibilities, e.g. selecting study subjects, obtaining consent, signing CRFs, making significant clinical assessments of the study subject during the study, etc.). Thus, it is important to design a signature page to capture all necessary signatures. It is not credible to have a protocol signature page requiring only the signature of the head of the department when he/she may never actually see patients. (The argument that the head of the department 'takes responsibility for all persons under her/his supervision' does not provide great confidence that those to whom responsibilities have been delegated are fully prepared.) For the safety of the study subject, the sponsor/CRO should be fully informed of specific site personnel to whom responsibilities have been delegated, and should require written evidence of their agreement to comply with the protocol. In our audit database, the responsible investigators, those actually managing the study and treating study subjects, did not sign the protocol at 27% of 378 study sites.

The protocol must be translated into the national language if the protocol is to be used in a country in which any site personnel are not sufficiently proficient in English (or whatever working language is in effect) or if the protocol is to be submitted to an ethics committee/IRB where it might be expected that some members are not sufficiently proficient in English. Thus, it is not a credible situation when English documents are observed at study sites where it is obvious that many personnel are not competent in the language.

To control distribution and approval of the protocol, copies of all signature pages, as well as a list of recipients, will be retained by the sponsor/CRO. Investigators (and any other signatories at study sites) should also keep a copy of the signature page. (A copy of anything signed should be retained by the signatories!)

Copies of all versions of the protocol will also be retained. It is critical that all versions are labelled and dated: in particular, the final approved document should be labelled as 'Final'.

The approved final protocol cannot be changed, except through the process of a formal protocol amendment procedure, described in Chapter 4. Thus, if further changes are required to an approved protocol by other external reviewers (e.g. ethics committees/IRBs or regulatory authorities), a formal protocol amendment procedure must be followed.

Obviously, study subjects must not receive any treatment before the protocol (and CRF) is finalised and approved by the sponsor/CRO, investigators, regulatory authorities and ethics committees/IRBs. However, in our audit database, study subjects received study treatment before the final protocol was approved at 18% of 378 sites.

2.2 CRFS AND OTHER DATA COLLECTION FORMS

Any document used to collect research data on clinical study subjects may be generically classed as a data collection form. These completed forms provide evidence of the research conducted. The most common type of data collection form is the case report form (CRF). Other types of data collection forms include diary cards, dispensing records, quality of life forms, etc. (Informed consent forms, subject registration forms and medication/device dispensing records are also data collection forms which might be prepared by the sponsor/CRO, but these documents must be treated differently because they are likely to contain patient names – this is considered further in Chapter 5.)

It is critical to ensure that data are collected in accordance with the protocol and must allow for proper analysis of the data and proper reporting of the data in the final clinical study report. CRFs must never require data that are not requested by the protocol and that will not be used in analyses: similarly, the CRF must capture all information requested by the protocol. The CRF must reflect the protocol exactly: no more and no less data must be collected. Thus, a CRF must be created for each clinical study and must be prepared in parallel with the protocol. Some guidelines for preparing CRFs are noted in Checklists 2.2–1 and 2.2–2. CRFs are usually prepared by sponsors/CROs in pharmaceutical industry research because of the demanding requirements for their design and contents.

... A study of an anticoagulant, Denmark, 13 patients
*The design of the CRF only required certain types of concomitant medications to be recorded. Although all patients were hospitalised and undergoing surgical procedures, the investigators were instructed not to collect any information on antiemtics, anxiolytics and antidiuretics. Also, events associated with acute myocardial infarction (e.g. angina, bundle branch block, asystole, ventricular tachycardia) were not reported as AEs as the CRF only requested this to be done if the events were considered to be **related** to study medication.* It is so difficult to eliminate bias in data collection. CRFs like these, instructing investigators not to report information which might be important for assessment of the study, do not help!

... A study of condition X, France, 22 patients
The CRF required HIV test results to be recorded. This was not required by the protocol. Neither the patients nor the ethics committee were aware that HIV testing was being conducted. The investigator also did not know this when the protocol was signed.
Clearly some data collection can be very sensitive and ethics committees/IRBs and prospective patients must be fully informed. A physician in the UK stated in one of our training meetings that even if cholesterol levels were measured and recorded in his clinical notes without his knowledge, he would object. He was concerned that insurance companies might have access to this information!

If CRF amendments are required (e.g. after review by ethics committees/IRBs), a formal amendment procedure must be followed and documented. Changes to CRFs may have an impact on the information sheet provided to study subjects and perhaps require that subjects give consent again.

Like the protocol, the CRF and especially any documents to be completed by study subjects, must obviously be translated into the local national language.

... A study of mortality of survivors of myocardial infarction, UK, 56 patients
The auditors found several CRF pages, describing details of AEs, which had not been retrieved by the monitor for over 12 months! This meant that the sponsor was not aware of the details of the safety data for this long time period. This evidently occurred because the CRF was designed to require a start date and a stop date for each safety event. For those events that were continuing, a stop date could not be recorded and so everyone agreed to wait until the end of the study before completing details of the event! The solution would have been to include a column in the CRF to record 'event continuing' so that the monitor could have retrieved the CRFs promptly.

... A study of an anxiolytic, France, 12 patients
The original English versions of psychiatric rating scales were translated into French by the local investigator and monitor. There was no system for verification of the translation. A formal translation procedure must be in place, particularly for documents such as these where comparability across study sites is so important.

Checklist 2.2–1. Information to be Collected in CRFs

The following basic information should be collected in all CRFs:
- Confirmation that consent has been obtained: both the date (and time) of providing information and the date (and time) on which the subject provided consent must be recorded;
- List of inclusion and exclusion criteria, in a checklist format;
- Baseline assessments: demographic data: date of birth, race (if this is considered to be a factor influencing response), sex, precautions against pregnancy, smoking habits or alcohol consumption, presenting condition, relevant history of condition, present and previous treatment; coexisting and previous conditions, general medical history, results of physical examination (e.g. height, weight, vital signs, primary diagnostic criteria);
- Dosing of study medications/devices (e.g. start date and end date for each treatment period, details of any unused material returned by subject at each visit, assessment of compliance, details of dose dispensed);
- Concomitant illnesses (diagnosis, duration, date of onset, intensity,

outcome), including diseases which were present before the study began and have persisted. (For conditions which begin after the start of the study, the information must be recorded in the AE section of the CRF.) Details of concomitant treatments (e.g. name, dose, start date, end date or indication of continuation date and reason) should be recorded. Details of medications/devices stopped prior to study treatment during a defined interval should also be recorded.

- Safety, including the nature, date of onset, continuation or stop date, action taken, outcome, frequency, severity, seriousness, and opinion of drug relationship. Scales for assessing severity and drug relationship must be provided. The means of soliciting AE information must be described. Serious AEs should be documented on a special form. For 'clinical laboratory data (e.g. clinical chemistry, haematology and urinalysis), only tests specified in the protocol should be listed. If any AEs require the investigator to break the treatment code in a double-blind study, this must also be recorded on the CRF.
- Effectiveness (e.g. efficacy, quality of life, economic benefit), including time, date and result of assessment; overall assessment of treatment (effectiveness and tolerance);
- Premature termination of study, including reason (e.g. side effects, other medical reasons, non medical reason, etc.), normal termination of the study, provision for follow-up assessments, if relevant (e.g. death report, autopsy report).

Checklist 2.2–2. Basic Design Features of CRFs

In designing CRFs, the following items should be considered:
- The cover page should include identifiers such as the sponsor/CRO name, identification of the study medication/device, title of study, study subject number/code, etc.
- Uniquely numbered to aid in accountability of all distributed CRFs;
- Divided into units (e.g. modules, booklets) corresponding to the data required for individual study visits (or groups of study visits if the visits are less than four–six weeks apart). This allows the monitor to retrieve a copy of the CRF unit that has been completed and signed by the investigator and to return the CRF unit to the sponsor/CRO for prompt data processing.

- Each page of the CRF booklet should be identified by the study code, visit identification, date (and time) of visit, date (and time) of assessment performance, subject initials, subject number and page number ('x of x pages') to ensure that all CRFs pages are returned to the sponsor/CRO. This will also help to ensure that the investigator uses the correct subject numbers when entering subjects into a clinical study, that subjects are entered in the correct order and that the investigator enters the prescribed number of subjects; for multicentre studies, space must be allowed to identify study sites on every page.
- Designed on three-part forms so that the sponsor/CRO receives the top copy (original) for archiving and the middle copy for use by data processing personnel. The investigator usually retains the bottom copy, which must be checked by the monitor at the study site to ensure that it is legible. Thin cardboard back copies or a cardboard insertion sheet must be used to ensure that entries are not copied to the wrong CRF pages. Single-page CRFs, requiring photocopying, are not acceptable.
- Comprising bound pages, not loose pages (except for SAE forms, diary cards, quality of life forms);
- Including a table of contents and a copy of the flow chart provided in the protocol. Instructions for completion of CRFs and correction of data entries must be an integral part of the CRF (not a separate document).
- Subject diaries, if applicable, should be designed to be easily used by the subject. A name, address and telephone number, must be provided for emergency contact if it is not provided on a separate card.

2.3   INVESTIGATOR BROCHURES

To ensure that an investigator is adequately informed and prepared for a clinical study of a new study medication/device, a current investigator brochure (or authorised summary of pre-study information) must be provided by the sponsor/CRO for review by all investigators. (If the study is to be conducted with a marketed product, the data sheet (or package insert, product monograph, etc) and any other new information (e.g. changes in the formulation or additional pharmacokinetic data) may be sufficient to adequately inform the investigator.)

The investigator must be given time to evaluate the contents of the brochure prior to approving the protocol and agreeing to conduct a clinical study, and of course the investigator brochure must be relevant and understandable to the investigator and other site personnel. In our audit database, no investigator brochures were evidently provided at 18% of 226 study sites. We advise investigators not to sign protocols until a current brochure is received.

Investigator brochures are usually prepared by sponsors (and more rarely by CROs), rather than investigators because the technical information in these documents is usually proprietary and confidential. Also, there are regulatory requirements which must be followed. In our audit database, many investigator brochures were not adequately comprehensive: the brochures we observed at 226 study sites were deficient in the following respects: no instructions for spills or wastage (85% of sites); no instructions for management of accidental exposure (50%); no summary of possible medication/device interactions (47%); no instructions for storage (47%); and no summary of contraindications and precautions (27%).

... A study of an anxiolytic, Germany, nine patients
The investigator brochure was provided to the study site six days after enrolment of the first patient. Obviously, the site personnel did not review details about the product prior to the study.

... A study involving cardiovascular surgery, Germany, 15 patients
The investigator brochure was not in the investigator site files. The investigator reported that he had loaned it to a colleague in another hospital.

... A study of prostate cancer, UK, 32 patients
An investigator brochure was not provided – the company argued that a brochure was unnecessary because the drug was marketed. It was – for hypertension! The protocol stated that safety and efficacy had been demonstrated: however, no evidence of supporting data were provided.

The investigator brochure must be current: at the very least, it should not be more than one year old. This requirement is particularly important because the brochure is a formal source of safety information. The contents of the investigator brochure must be reviewed at least annually by the sponsor/CRO, or as new significant information (e.g. new safety data) becomes available. Some significant new information (e.g. fatal or life-threatening events) should be immediately transmitted to all investigators and the investigator brochure must be updated as soon as possible thereafter. In our database, we observed that the brochure provided at the start of the study was not current at 30% of 226 investigator sites, and at 33% of the sites, the brochure was not updated during the study.

... A study of antifungal treatment, UK, 29 patients
The investigator brochure predated the study by five years and indicated that there were no AEs at all associated with treatment. In theory, all AEs reported should have been labelled as 'unexpected'. We are always suspicious of claims of no adverse events – this would be unusual for any medication/device.

... A study of hypertension, Germany, 32 patients
The investigator brochure predated the study by nine years.

Investigator brochures will be used by external individuals (e.g. investigators, other site personnel, ethics committees/ IRBs and regulatory authorities) and these individuals must all be instructed to treat the document confidentially because it contains proprietary information. Prompt return of the investigator brochure will be requested if the investigator is unable to conduct a proposed study. To control distribution and help maintain confidentiality, a list of investigator brochure recipients containing the recipient's name, address, number of copies sent and received, investigator brochure date and the date sent will be maintained by the sponsor/CRO. This list must also indicate details of returns and destruction of superseded copies. When investigator brochures are reissued, the superseded versions must be recovered. However, the investigator should always retain one copy of the superseded version at the study site so that there is evidence of the information which was available to the investigator at the time he or she was conducting the study.

... A study of hormone replacement therapy, France, 19 patients
The investigator brochure was in English, although the investigator
could not communicate in English with the auditors.

2.4   REGULATORY REQUIREMENTS

Regulatory authority review and/or approval is usually necessary in all countries before, during and after clinical studies, although there are some exceptions (e.g. Phase I studies in the UK). No medications or devices should be sent to study sites before regulatory authorisation. This is a specialised area, usually handled by the sponsor/CRO, rather than the investigator, and a few brief comments are only included here to help clinical research personnel understand some requirements (Checklist 2.4–1). Usually, a group known as the 'regulatory affairs department', part of the sponsor/CRO, handles regulatory submissions.

Normally, as part of the submission, there must be an indication that studies are conducted in the context of a clinical plan, often referred to as a clinical development plan. The regulators wish to know that studies are being conducted for good reason – study subjects must not be exposed to risk unnecessarily – and not simply for marketing purposes. Thus, there must be a clinical development plan which is a formal document for describing the overall strategy for the development of the medication/device. The plan will describe the extent and objectives of clinical studies which are necessary for development of products so as to expose the minimum number of subjects to the risks of clinical studies. Unless a copy of the approved development plan is required for regulatory purposes or inspection, it should normally be treated as a confidential internal company document and should not be distributed to any investigators (actual or potential), consultants or other outside parties. However, all parties, including study subjects, should receive an adequate answer to the question – why is the study being conducted?

Checklist 2.4–1. Items to be Submitted to Regulatory Authorities

The following items should be submitted to regulatory authorities, depending on local regulations, before studies begin:

- Identity of sponsor/CRO; CVs of sponsor/CRO personnel;
- Overall clinical development plan; evidence of approval, authorisations, refusals, suspensions or withdrawals in other countries;
- Information about all medications/devices to be used in the study. (Special consideration needs to be given to comparator products not licensed in the country where the study is being conducted.)
- Sites used for assembly or packaging of product. (Special consideration also needs to be given to activities such as encapsulation for blinding purposes or dissolution testing); identity of manufacturer, if this is other than the sponsor/CRO; identity of importer, if applicable; special requirements for certain types of products (e.g. medications of biological origin, radio-labelled products, biotechnology products);
- Sample study medication/device labels;
- Investigator brochure (or other preclinical summary) and any publications;
- Title and phase of studies, and objectives of research;
- Planned start-up date for studies with proposed duration;
- Protocols, CRFs; informed consent forms and information sheets;
- Ethics committee/IRB approvals (and rejections, if any), if available at the time of the submission. If not, it may be necessary to submit them at a later date, depending on local regulations.
- List of proposed investigators with addresses, CVs; identity and details of CRO, financial arrangements with investigators (e.g. in France); permission of institute in which research will be conducted (e.g. in France); insurance provisions;
- Clinical laboratory certification and reference ranges.

2.5   SELECTION OF INVESTIGATORS AND STUDY SITES

The sponsor/CRO has a duty to place a study safely – that is, only qualified investigators and suitable facilities must be selected. The sponsor/CRO must go through a formal assessment procedure before placement of a study.

... A study of an anxiolytic, several sites in Europe
Study medication was issued to eight investigators before any assessment visits by the sponsor. This is not a rare finding. The

sponsors/CROs always seem to be surprised in these situations when things do not work out as expected!

Potential suitable investigators and study sites may be identified by several means, such as a review of previous experience with the sponsor or CRO, recommendations by colleagues and other investigators, review of literature, contacts during professional meetings, and reputation (e.g. an opinion leader in the field of interest).

If a decision is made at this point to proceed further, a confidentiality agreement will be issued, signed and received by the sponsor/CRO, before confidential details are disclosed. The protocol and CRF (which may be in draft form at this stage), the proposed information sheet/consent form, and the investigator brochure may be sent to the investigator for review prior to a pre-study assessment visit, and after receipt from the investigator of a signed confidentiality agreement:

If the outcome of preliminary discussions is satisfactory, a curriculum vitae (CV) (or résumé) of all investigators at the study site, substantiating the investigators' qualifications to conduct a clinical study, should be requested and can be collected at the pre-study assessment visit. If the potential investigator is considered suitable, a formal pre-study assessment visit will be organised by the sponsor/CRO. An agenda should be organised in advance, stating who will need to be available during the assessment, and which facilities will be assessed.

If the investigator and facilities are known to the sponsor/CRO (i.e. a study has previously been conducted with the site under consideration), a pre-study assessment visit is still necessary to determine that there have been no significant changes at the study site since the previous study was completed. In all cases, a pre-study visit assessment cannot be replaced by a meeting with the investigator alone or by an initiation meeting, since a full assessment of facility and staff adequacy is dependent on first-hand observation obtained only by a site visit. (It is extremely important at this stage to find out how much the investigator is currently doing and whether or not he/she is truly interested in the study. Separate visits to the clinical laboratory and the contract research organisation may be necessary.) Checklists 2.5–1 and 2.5–2 provide some guidance on what must be reviewed during these assessment visits.

... During the debriefing after an audit, an investigator in a London hospital whispered to one of five nursing sisters at the meeting: 'Which study are we talking about?'

... A study of back pain, UK, 29 patients
Supplies for at least nine other studies involving eight different companies were openly available on the shelves in the investigator's office. He was a general practitioner and worked independently. Any experienced monitor knows that a quick glance around the investigator's office will provide clues about workload. This example, and some noted below, should cause the 'red warning flag' to go up.

... A study of an inhaler for asthma, UK, 12 patients
The auditors observed evidence in the investigator's office (e.g. CRFs) showing involvement in more than 25 different studies.

... A study of hypertension, Canada, 15 patients
The auditors referred to this site as 'the factory'. Patients were shifted from one study to another in sequence: in one case, the washout period between studies was one day. One patient had participated in 12 different studies over a 15-year period. This example also illustrates why it is so important that the subject's notes should indicate their participation in studies. How safe was this setting for study subjects?

... A study of coronary artery disease, Northern Ireland, 16 patients
The study started in April 199x. In March 199x, the investigator had written that he would not have time for the study. In fact, the study was conducted by other physicians, but none of these were declared as investigators in the protocol or any other documentation. Monitors must determine from the beginning exactly who will be conducting the study. There is no point in having senior investigators sign documents and attend briefing meetings rather than their colleagues who are actually doing the work.

... A study of cardiovascular surgery, USA, 47 patients
The auditors observed a letter to the sponsor from the investigator indicating that he thought the study design was biased in favour of the sponsor's drug. The company responded, but the investigator was still

not convinced and expressed this strongly in writing. He carried on with the study anyway!

... A study of an anxiolytic, several sites in Europe
This study employed psychiatrists in Germany, general practitioners in France and nurses in UK. (Although general practitioners were listed as investigators in the UK, nurses were actually conducting all psychiatric assessments.) The study was eventually abandoned, after several hundred patients were recruited, because of too much variation between study sites. Clearly, this is unfair to the study subjects who had gone through the risk of a clinical study for nothing.

... A study of allergies, Germany, two sites, 44 patients
At one site, one of the study subjects was an investigator; at another site, one of the study subjects was the study site co-ordinator. She was also conducting the skin tests on all other patients.

After the pre-study assessment visit, the monitor will document the discussions and findings and prepare a detailed pre-study assessment visit report. If the site is considered to be acceptable after the pre-study assessment visit, arrangements should be made for an initiation visit to brief all the staff associated with the study, as a group, if possible. In the case of a multicentre study, arrangements for the start-up meeting (group meeting of all investigators) must also be organised.

If the investigator is not selected for the study, all items which may have been previously sent to the investigator must be retrieved to maintain confidentiality.

Checklist 2.5–1. Items to Consider at Pre-Study Assessment Visits

The following items should be assessed at study sites by sponsor/CRO monitors at pre-study assessment visits:
- Study site personnel: availability of study staff; specific allocation of responsibilities (e.g. study co-ordination, storage/dispensing of study materials, randomisation of study subjects, treatment allocation, completion of CRFs, collection and storage of samples, assessment of study subjects at each routine visit, recruitment,

screening and evaluation, scheduling of study subject visits and follow-up); how long study co-ordinator has been at the site; workload of the study co-ordinator during a given week; clinic days; schedule of investigator; availability of investigator and other representatives to attend investigator start-up meeting and meet with monitor during monitoring visits.

- Facilities: offices, wards, archives, pharmacy, clinical laboratory, study medication/device storage areas; environmental control maintenance of factors such as temperature, light and humidity; backup storage area in case of power loss; disaster recovery scheme; alert system for disaster; inventory control procedures; separate storage for investigational study supplies; time during which pharmacist is on duty, availability if not 24 hours; designated research pharmacist; security of storage; dispensing procedures for outpatients; provision of instruction in medication/device use; labelling; control of medication/device in inpatient studies; accountability procedures; maintaining records of receipt and shipment; name and address of the clinical laboratory and determination of quality assurance systems of the clinical laboratory (e.g. evidence of accreditation, certification, participation in proficiency testing, maintenance and control of analysers); provision of signed and dated copy of laboratory reference ranges; access to source documents; ethics committee/IRB requirements (e.g. membership, waiting period for meetings, documentation to submit for meetings);

- Suitable study subject population: access to suitable subjects in sufficient numbers; how subjects will be recruited; source (e.g. from investigator's subject population or be referred by other physicians); if referred, means by which investigator will obtain adequate evidence of medical history; use of advertisements; potential subject enrolment (recruitment) rate. The monitor must obtain documented evidence (e.g. anonymised computer printout of patients in clinical setting) to substantiate the proposed recruitment of eligible study subjects.

- Monitoring procedures: the monitor must ensure that there is agreement on the frequency and nature of contacts (e.g. telephone or fax), availability of the investigator and other site personnel during visits, available working area; and access to other facilities (e.g. pharmacy, clinical laboratory).

Checklist 2.5–2. Additional Considerations for Assessment of Phase I Facilities

Assessment of Phase I facilities should address the following items, in addition to those normally reviewed:

- Adequate source of volunteers and sufficiently large volunteer panel, considering the following: access to special populations (e.g. elderly, postmenopausal women, renally impaired patients, hepatically impaired patients, depressed patients, etc.); and procedures to inform primary care physicians of study participation;
- Staff with experience in the following: clinical pharmacology and pharmacokinetics; venepuncture, diets and standardised meals; technical expertise to handle biological samples; drug-of-abuse testing, ability to perform analyses at night or during weekends; qualified pharmacist for preparation and dispensing study medication/device;
- Adequate facilities, including the following: facilities for handling and storage (long-term) of biological samples; rooms for pharmacodynamic measurements; central clock in study rooms; cleaning facilities; computerised data management system which controls sample movements; facilities to prepare labels for tubes; facilities for leisure activities; screening rooms; showers and toilets; laboratory rooms; kitchen for supply of standardised meals; and adequate number of beds (typically 12);
- Safety and emergency equipment and procedures, including: emergency drug supplies; oxygen; suction; defribillator with ECG monitor; continuous ECG monitors with arrhythmia detection; endotracheal tubes; stretchers; wheelchair; pumps for intravenous administration; alarm system to locate the sites of emergencies; and staff skilled in resuscitation;
- Suitable location considering: access by public transport and proximity to a general hospital with emergency room.

2.6   QUALIFICATIONS OF CLINICAL RESEARCH PERSONNEL

All clinical research personnel (sponsor/CRO and study site) must be appropriately qualified, experienced, and trained prior to undertaking assigned tasks in the management of clinical studies.

For site personnel, many others beside investigators (e.g. study site co-ordinators , research nurses, pharmacists, laboratory personnel) may need to provide evidence of qualifications for their role in the study. However, all studies involving research of investigational medications and devices require qualified investigators. The internationally accepted standard for 'qualified' includes three main criteria: medically qualified, that is, legally licensed to practice medicine as a physician; experienced in the relevant therapeutic speciality; and experienced in clinical research. We tend to avoid terms such as 'co-investigator', 'sub-investigator', 'associate investigator', 'principal investigator', and 'assistant investigator': during audits, we simply try to determine who is actually undertaking investigator responsibilities and then we expect documentation of their qualifications to act as investigators.

Investigators (and other site personnel) will be asked to submit documented evidence of their qualifications by providing a CV and any other supporting documentation to the sponsor/CRO. These are usually assessed by monitors and retained in the study files. Obviously, the information in CVs and other evidence obtained at the assessment visits should be reviewed carefully. Our audit database indicated that the documentation was deficient at 226 study sites in the following respects: no indication of investigator training in GCP (86%); no indication of other clinical research commitments (64%); no indication of availability of time for the study (65%); CVs were not signed (47%); no indication of usual responsibilities (42%); CV did not indicate previous experience in clinical research (40%); and CVs were not dated (28%).

... A study of cardiovascular surgery, Sweden, 12 patients
The investigator's CV indicated that he was working and living in Texas, USA. The study was being conducted in Sweden!

Evidence of sponsor/CRO personnel qualifications should also be available. These are normally retained by the sponsor/CRO only, not the investigators. The following evidence should be retained: a file of qualifications and experience which documents educational qualifications (e.g. degrees, diplomas, certificates, etc) and prior employment experience and which should be revised whenever there are new significant achievements (e.g. attainment of a new degree, experience in a different therapeutic area, etc.); a training record which documents items such as presentations, seminars, courses, lectures, in-house reviews, etc. which have been undertaken by the employee during the employment period with the sponsor/CRO; an organisation chart which must be dated and include the names and titles of employees, demonstrating reporting and working relationships; and generic job descriptions. All evidence pertaining to qualifications, experience, training and supervision should be available for scrutiny by inspectors and therefore should not contain personal or confidential information (e.g. salary) which will be maintained in a separate personnel file. In our auditing experience, sponsor/CRO files are missing important information in several areas with respect to sponsor/CRO training: no monitor CVs (75% of 226 sites); no evidence of training in SOPs (57%); no evidence of training in the therapeutic area (53%); no evidence of training in GCP (36%); and no evidence of adequate experience (29%).

All sponsor/CRO personnel in clinical research will be expected to undertake external or in-house training (courses, conferences, workshops) which is relevant to the implementation of GCP. Personnel must be trained in current SOPs and must regularly review, update and discuss the current clinical research as part of the training. Consideration should be given to training in the therapeutic area, limited GLP and GMP requirements, data management, regulatory affairs, statistics, management techniques, communications skills, etc. Personnel training files will be revised whenever new significant training programmes are undertaken (e.g. training in a particular therapeutic area).

Specimen signature lists, which also indicate responsibilities, should be initiated and maintained for both sponsor/CRO and study site personnel.

2.7   STUDY AGREEMENTS

Many contracts or agreements must be prepared, understood and authorised before clinical studies begin. The most obvious ones include: the protocol and case report form; a list of investigator responsibilities (often in addition to the protocol); finances; confidentiality; insurance/indemnity; and contracts between the sponsor and the CRO.

The investigator must conduct clinical research in accordance with the protocol. The formal agreement of the investigator to abide by the specified policies should be obtained in writing and all investigators (e.g. any physicians who undertake investigator responsibilities for the study such as assessing study subjects, signing CRFs, obtaining consent, changing dosing, assessing AEs, etc.) and representatives of the sponsor/CRO must sign the final study protocol to indicate agreement with the contents. If a 'principal' investigator is designated at the study site, the protocol must also be signed by any other physicians undertaking investigator responsibilities (e.g. co-investigators, sub-investigators, assistant investigators, associate investigators, etc.).

A separate investigator agreement, specifying all responsibilities is usually necessary, in addition to the protocol, to emphasize certain aspects of the protocol. (This is because protocols are lengthy detailed documents and the main responsibilities may not be apparent.) This agreement should also be signed by each investigator who signs the protocol, unless a principal investigator is declared and the agreement specifically refers to all investigators, and must also be signed by representatives of the sponsor/CRO. It should be signed and agreed after the site assessment visit, but before the initiation meeting. In multicentre studies, an agreement must be available for each study centre. The responsibilities agreement should also highlight sponsor/CRO responsibilities with regard to provision of materials (e.g. study medications/devices, CRFs, equipment). Checklists 2.7–1 and 2.7–2 highlight some of the main investigator and sponsor/CRO responsibilities, respectively.

... A study of an anticoagulant, Italy, 19 patients
The formal agreement for the study was not finalised until seven months after recruitment had been ongoing.

A study may not start and confidential material may not be released before a confidentiality agreement is agreed and signed. Confidential information (e.g. any proprietary information of the sponsor/CRO) may only be revealed to site personnel directly involved in the study. Other site personnel besides the investigator (e.g. site co-ordinator, pharmacist) may also be required to sign confidentiality agreements if they are receiving confidential information. Of course, all parties must respect confidentiality.

... A study being conducted in Italy by a large multinational company
While reviewing the sponsor affiliate files, the auditors came across a copy of a complete protocol from another company in the same thera-peutic area. The protocol had apparently been obtained from a UK monitor who had been given the protocol by an investigator. A memo was attached to this protocol, indicating that it was distributed inter-nationally. The memo directed all recipients to note the names of the investigators and the progress of the 'competitor'. Was this a case of industrial espionage?

Insurance for protection of study subjects and indemnity for investigators and institutions is mandatory in many countries where clinical studies are performed. The sponsor/CRO must determine the local requirements to provide adequate insurance. Information regarding compensation must be available to any subject in a clinical study, whether or not compensation is provided – in the USA, in particular, compensation may not be available – and must be communicated to study subjects in the information sheet and the consent form. The investigator, study subjects, clinical institutions (e.g. hospitals), and ethics commit-tees/IRBs must also be notified of insurance terms. The sponsor/CRO is responsible for ensuring that insurance coverage stays current throughout the study and all personnel should be aware that protocol amendments and updates of inves-tigator brochures may require review of insurance agreements.

... A study of allergies, Germany, 12 patients
The name of the insurance company on the information sheet provided to study subjects was different from that in the protocol.

... A study of hormone replacement therapy, Canada, 13 study subjects
The protocol referred to the ABPI guidelines. Many documents refer

to guidelines which are probably never available to the investigator or to the study subjects. The ABPI is the Association for the British Pharmaceutical Industry – not relevant at all to Canada!

Items to consider in financial agreements are noted in Checklist 2.7–3. Financial agreements must also specify the terms in which payment will not be made (e.g. data cannot be used because they are incorrect, illegible, incomplete, etc.). In multicentre studies, a financial agreement must be available for each site and the costs for each site or subject in a multicentre study should be comparable. The final payment should not be made until the study has been satisfactorily completed in accordance with the financial agreement. The schedule of payments to investigators must be agreed and the monitor must check that there is compliance with the schedule. The financial agreement should specify the event that will trigger a payment (e.g. submission of an invoice or inclusion or completion of a specific number of patients. Payments to study subjects (e.g. in Phase I studies) may have implications for tax and this must be considered at the beginning of the study.

... A study of dyspepsia, UK, 32 subjects
The financial agreement covered eight subjects – 32 were recruited. This was not only a financial problem. Was the ethics committee informed? Why were four times as many subjects recruited as planned? What was the impact on other sites? What are the statistical implications for the study?

... A study of an anticoagulant, Australia, 26 patients
The financial agreement (which also specified many of the investigator's responsibilities) was not finalised until eight months after the initiation of the study.

Checklist 2.7–1. Investigator Responsibilities

The following investigator responsibilities must be declared in agreements or contracts:

- Adhere to the protocol exactly. No changes to the protocol may be undertaken without following a formal protocol amendment procedure and without agreement by the sponsor/CRO.
- Be thoroughly familiar with the properties of the clinical study medications/devices as described in the investigator brochure;
- Have sufficient time to personally conduct and complete the study. If more than one investigator is involved at a specific study site, the specific responsibilities must be described for each investigator. The investigator must ensure that no other studies divert study subjects, facilities or personnel from the study under consideration.
- Maintain the confidentiality of all information received with regard to the study and the investigational study medication/device;
- Submit the protocol, information sheet and consent form, and other required documentation, to an ethics committee/IRB for review and approval before the study begins. During the study, the investigator is also responsible for submitting any new information (e.g. protocol amendments, safety information) which might be important for continuing risk assessment by the ethics committee/IRB.
- Obtain informed consent from each study subject prior to enrolment into the study;
- Inform the subject's primary care physician (e.g. general practitioner or family physician) of proposed study participation before enrolment into the study;
- Maintain study subject clinical notes (i.e. source documents) separately from the CRFs. The source documents must support the data entered into the CRFs and must clearly indicate participation in a clinical study. If the study subject is referred by another physician, the investigator must ensure that sufficient evidence is available in the clinical notes to support the eligibility of the study subject;
- Maintain a confidential list identifying the number/code and names of all subjects entered into the study;
- Allow authorised representatives of the sponsor/CRO and regulatory authorities direct access to study subject clinical notes (source documents) in order to verify the data recorded on CRFs;
- Ensure CRFs are complete and accurate;
- Allow monitoring visits by the sponsor/CRO at a predetermined frequency. During these monitoring visits, the monitor must be allowed to communicate with all site personnel involved in the conduct of the clinical study;

- Report all AEs and SAEs to the sponsor/CRO and follow the special reporting requirements for SAEs;
- Maintain the security and accountability of clinical study supplies, ensure that medications/devices are labelled properly, maintain records of clinical study medication/device dispensing, including dates, quantity and use by study subjects; and return or disposition (as instructed by the sponsor/CRO) after completion or termination of the study;
- Archive all CRFs and documents associated with the study for a minimum of 15 years. Notify the sponsor/CRO of any problems with archiving in potential unusual circumstances (e.g. investigator retires, relocates, dies; study subject dies, relocates, etc.);
- Provide reports of the study's progress whenever required;
- Review the final clinical report, and sign and date the signature page after review;
- Allow an independent audit and/or inspection of all study documents and facilities;
- Agree to the publication policy;
- Agree to the sponsor/CRO's ownership of the data;
- Agree to the stated time frames for the study (e.g. start and completion of recruitment, submission of completed CRFs);
- Work to GCP as defined by the ICH, FDA and local regulations. These must be clearly described to the investigator.

Checklist 2.7–2. Sponsor/CRO Responsibilities

The following sponsor/CRO responsibilities should be clearly declared in contracts or agreements:
- Provide all necessary materials (e.g. study medications/devices, CRFs, equipment, etc.);
- Provide the investigators, other site personnel, the ethics committee/ IRB (not directly but through the investigator), and the regulatory authority, with all necessary information and provide regular updates with particular reference to issues about the safety of the study medications/devices;
- If equipment is only loaned, this must be specified with an indication of when it will be retrieved by the sponsor/CRO and who is responsible for maintenance and calibration;
- Ensure frequent and thorough monitoring of the study;

- Ensure that the study is conducted in accordance with the protocol, and any amendments;
- Maintain adequate records showing the receipt, shipment, use or other disposition of the study medication or device;
- Retain documentation for the required time period;
- Provide adequate insurance for the protection of the study subject, and indemnity for the investigators and the institution.

Checklist 2.7–3. Items in Financial Agreements

Financial agreements between sponsors/CROs and site personnel should address the following items:
- Fees for services, provided that the cost of the services is not paid from another source. The sponsor/CRO will negotiate, with the investigator, the costs per subject or the total amount. If costs are based on visits, or completion of certain stages of the study, these must be specified in the financial agreement.
- Salaries of support staff, provided that they are not paid from another source;
- Small items of equipment;
- Expendables such as syringes, catheters and dressings, etc.
- Study subject costs, e.g. travel (taxi, bus);
- Advertising costs, if any, for recruitment of subjects;
- Institutional overheads, if any;
- Attendance of staff at scientific or educational meetings;
- Ethics committee/IRB fee, if applicable.

2.8   SELECTION OF CROs

CROs may be used for many different services (e.g. monitoring, writing, auditing, data management, biostatistics, etc.) and the proportion of research assigned to CROs has increased dramatically in the last decade. The policy of the sponsor must be to select CROs which work in conformance with the current international standards of GCP and therefore a careful evaluation of a candidate CRO must be performed prior to placing an assignment. Checklists 2.8–1 and 2.8–2 provide some guidance on the selection of CROs and subsequent contractual agreements.

After placement, further management of the CRO is necessary

to ensure the progress of the study in a timely and efficient manner. It is usually the responsibility of a sponsor monitor or project manager to maintain contact with the CRO on a regular and frequent basis (at least weekly) to ensure that the study is being conducted in accordance with the contract. The monitor will record observations about the conduct of the CRO during the study in monitor reports. Any deficiencies observed in the conduct of the study will be reported immediately in writing to senior sponsor personnel, to determine any corrective action required.

... A phase I study, Europe, 15 study subjects
A study had been conducted by a CRO for Company X. During the audit, the auditors noted a handwritten comment on a CRO letter indicating that the results should not be published as they showed the product to be better than that of the comparator drug. The comparator drug was a product of another large client of the CRO.

... A study of an anticoagulant, Denmark, 13 patients and Australia, 26 patients
The local CROs conducting the study had no SOPs. We continue to be astonished that sponsors could hire CROs without confirming the presence of SOPs.

Checklist 2.8–1. Items to Review in Selecting CROs

In selecting CROs, the sponsor should review the following items:
- SOPs: quality of SOPs, compliance with SOPs, other QA systems (e.g. internal auditing, proficiency testing), and determine exactly which SOPs (i.e. sponsor or CRO) will be used;
- Range of services, reputation, experience in therapeutic area to be studied, previous experience with sponsor;
- Personnel (details of qualifications, training, experience, workloads and specific assignment for the study);
- Suitable facilities, equipment and technical ability for specific tests to be undertaken in the study, location (proximity and ease of access to study subjects and investigators), security, archiving, facilities for prompt communication with the sponsor and the study sites;

- Confidentiality provisions;
- Protocol and CRF development;
- Ethics committee(s) review and approval;
- Regulatory requirements;
- Monitoring standards/frequency;
- AE reporting procedures;
- Study medication/device management: packaging, labelling, storage, accountability and reconciliation, destruction or final disposition;
- Clinical laboratory requirements;
- Data management and statistical analysis, capability for data transfer, if needed, documentation of validation of computer systems;
- Clinical report production.

Checklist 2.8–2. Contracts with CROs

The contracts between CROs and sponsors should specify the following:
- Allocation of responsibilities;
- Monitoring strategy;
- Project timing;
- Reference to specific guidelines and regulations;
- Description of legislative jurisdiction;
- Provisions for amendments to the contract;
- Time period during which the contract is valid;
- Requirements for documentation (e.g. format, frequency) of all activities;
- Specific contact names;
- Confidentiality;
- Financial arrangements (including timing and condition under which payments will or will not be made).

2.9 SELECTING CLINICAL LABORATORIES

Almost all studies require clinical laboratory data to be collected. Sponsors and CROs must decide at the beginning of a study whether to use the local clinical laboratory or a central laboratory. There are advantages and disadvantages to both choices, but overall, sponsors seem to feel more confident with central laboratories, especially for large multicentre multinational studies.

Checklist 2.9–1 provide some guidance on selection of clinical laboratories. The responsibilities agreed must be clearly stated in a detailed contract. In addition to the items noted in Checklist 2.8–2 (contracts with CROs), the following should also be considered: specific tests to be undertaken and specific equipment and analysis procedures.

Before the studies begin, the sponsor/CRO must provide the clinical laboratory with: contact details for each investigator and study site and for the sponsor/CRO monitor. Contact numbers must be available on a 24-hour basis. The monitor should arrange for attendance of clinical laboratory personnel at multicentre start-up meetings (or individual site initiation visits) to demonstrate use of all items for the collection, storage and shipment of biological samples and the management of clinical laboratory reports.

Monitors must also work with the clinical laboratory to ensure that appropriate information is provided to investigators such as: routine and special procedures or equipment for collecting, handling, storing, packaging and shipping clinical samples; sample request forms with instructions for completion; labels with instructions for use; procedures to report test results; procedures for clinically significant results; and contact names and addresses for the clinical laboratory.

Checklist 2.9–1. Selecting Clinical Laboratories

In selecting clinical laboratories, sponsors/CROs should review the following items:

- SOPs: quality of SOPs, compliance with SOPs, other QA systems (e.g. proficiency testing, external quality assessments, accreditation and/or certification schemes traceable to national or international standards, and internal quality control);
- Range of services, reputation, evidence of laboratory certification and the licence number of the laboratory, previous experience with the sponsor/CRO;
- Personnel (details of qualifications, training, experience, workloads and specific assignment for the study);

- Suitable facilities, equipment and technical ability for specific tests to be undertaken in the study, location (proximity and ease of access to study subjects and investigators), security, archiving, confidentiality provisions; documentation of validation of computer systems; systems for prompt communication with the sponsor/CRO and the study sites, data management and capability for data transfer, if needed, equipment and technical ability for specific tests to be undertaken in the study, list of maintenance programmes, list of procedures for calibration or standardisation of equipment);
- Standardised (referenced) methods of conducting test procedures; standardised (referenced) methods and validation procedures for drug assay analyses, if applicable;
- Preparation of clinical laboratory protocol;
- Procedures for receipt of samples; storage facilities for samples; sampling kits. (Examine preparation, storage, distribution, labelling, accountability and reconciliation procedures.)
- Format of laboratory reports. (Obtain copies of sample request forms, labels, laboratory reports and ensure that reports include time/date of collection, shipment, receipt, analysis, and issue of report.)
- Reference ranges appropriate to study subject populations. A range is needed for each test. The sponsor/CRO should also assess: alert values, alarm values, panic values, cutoff values, special values needed for certain types of studies (e.g. cancer studies), identify units to be used and procedures for transformation of units, which values will trigger safety event reporting and procedures for obtaining standardised reporting from investigators with regard to assessment of out-of-range values.

2.10   INITIATION VISITS

Initiation visits must be distinguished from selection visits – the former occur after the site has been formally selected and before study subject enrolment. Basically, the sponsor/CRO undertakes initiation visits to ensure that nothing has changed since the previous visit, to confirm items previously discussed and retrieve missing documents for the sponsor/CRO archives, to demonstrate use of CRFs and the study medication/device, and to ensure that the investigator staff are co-ordinated in their activities (Checklists 2.10–1 and 2.10–2).

The initial briefing at a study site should be done at a formal study initiation meeting(s) at which the monitor and/ or other qualified sponsor/CRO representatives present details of the conduct of the study to the investigator and all appropriate staff. This provides an opportunity for the site personnel to collectively resolve any problems related with the study. The investigator may not enrol subjects until ethics committee/IRB approval has been obtained in writing and a study initiation visit has been conducted and study medications/devices will also not be delivered until this point. After the initiation visit, the monitor will prepare a report of all activities. The investigator may or may not receive a copy of this document, although we recommend providing copies as this is a helpful document for the site personnel. In our audit database, we have noted many deficiencies in initiation reports. In a sample of 226 sites, the initiation reports did not indicate review of the following items: archiving requirements (51%); investigator brochures (41%); procedures for breaking randomisation codes, if relevant (35%); GCP requirements (34%); investigator responsibilities (31%); clinical laboratory requirements (28%); and monitoring requirements (26%). The place of the initiation visit was not recorded on visit reports at 34% of 226 sites!

If the study is a multicentre study, a study start-up meeting of all investigators should take place prior to subject enrolment. A start-up meeting is not synonymous with an initiation meeting which must occur at each individual site and a start-up meeting may not substitute for an initiation meeting and vice versa. The objectives of the startup meeting are to present the protocol, discuss items to achieve a common understanding and consider standardisation requirements and to discuss and clarify practical details. Invitations to the start-up meeting should be extended to other site personnel (e.g. study co-ordinator, pharmacist) and the agenda, attendance, and minutes of the proceedings of the start-up meeting must be documented by the sponsor/CRO. According to our audit database, in a sample of 210 study sites involving multicentre studies, the investigators' attendance at a start-up meeting was not recorded at 33% of sites. Investigators at 25% of the sites were apparently not invited to a start-up meeting.

Checklist 2.10–1. Items to be Addressed at Study Initiation Visits

At study site initiation visits, the sponsor/CRO monitor will address the following items:

- Detailed review of the protocol and the requirement to follow the protocol exactly;
- Overall review of the study medication/device, handling and prescribing study medication/device, and procedures associated with the randomisation and blinding of medications/devices. A certain quantity of the medication/device must be available at the time of the initiation visit so that the monitor can verify receipt and to explain management of the supplies to the site personnel. If supplies are not available at this visit, the monitor must arrange another visit. Study subjects cannot be enrolled until study medications/devices have been checked by the monitor. The monitor must check the storage area, and check that there has been no breakage or inappropriate storage during shipment.
- Completion and management of CRFs, requirements for timely submission of CRFs (specify time), and requirements for source documents;
- Arrangements with clinical laboratories, pharmacies, wards, etc. The monitor should review procedures for handling specimens and ensure that sample collection kits have arrived safely in sufficient quantity.
- Obtaining of subject informed consent, submissions to ethics committees/IRBs during the study;
- Procedure for reporting AEs;
- Proposed schedule for monitoring and the need for access to source documents;
- Requirement to retain records securely for specified time periods.

Checklist 2.10–2. Items to be Provided to the Study Site Before the Study Begins

Before study subjects are enrolled, the sponsor/CRO monitor will ensure that site personnel have the following items:

- Current investigator brochure;
- Protocol (signed) and protocol amendments (signed), if applicable;
- Other signed agreements (e.g. confidentiality agreement, financial

agreement, letters of indemnity and insurance, investigator responsibilities agreement);

- Sufficient study medication/device to start the study, randomisation code list or codebreak envelopes, as appropriate, study medication/device shipment and receipt forms, and study medication/device accountability forms (for recording inventory, dispensing and returns);
- Sufficient CRFs, subject information sheets and consent forms and any other information to be provided to subjects (e.g. diary cards); serious AE report forms;
- Regulatory notification/approval documentation, as appropriate, evidence of marketing authorizations in other countries, information on any restrictions imposed by the regulatory authority (or the ethics committee/IRB);
- Guidelines for GCP;
- Special equipment (if required);
- Ethics committee/IRB review and approval letter, details of the working procedures of the ethics committee, membership list;
- Investigator CV and/or other statement of qualifications, CVs and training records (or other evidence of qualifications) of all site staff members involved in the study;
- Pre-study correspondence and assessment reports;
- Clinical laboratory reference ranges (signed and dated), clinical laboratory certification/accreditation.

CASE STUDY TWO

A Multicentre Double-Blind Placebo-Controlled Study to Assess the Efficacy and Safety of Drug X in the Treatment of Headache in Approximately 50 Study Subjects (USA).

During this audit, it was not hard to determine that investigator responsibilities were being delegated to whomever happened to be available. In fact, the auditors did not meet with the investigator during the audit: they were informed, a few days before the audit, that the investigator was available for a conference call for about 30–45 minutes. Apparently, during the study, he was only physically present in the clinic once every two weeks. The sponsor was not aware of the extent of delegation in this study.

Summary of Major Deficiencies

Standard Operating Procedures: Some important topics were not covered by the SOPs of the CRO (e.g. selection and management of other CROs for subcontracted data management, medication packaging etc; liaison with sponsors; financial payments to study subjects; source data verification procedures; preparation of CRFs for data processing; study medication/device control at the study site; and auditing).

IRB Review: Approval was not obtained from a local IRB. (In fact the reviewing IRB was several hundred miles away – the reviewing IRB could not really assess the local facilities or population.) Documentation for the local IRB had been prepared by the investigator and had been submitted to the IRB. However, this application was eventually withdrawn and this was not explained in the study documentation. There was no evidence that the local IRB was aware that a distant IRB had actually approved the study or that the study was being conducted.

The distant IRB was informed that the investigator and the 'sub-investigator' would be obtaining consent: in fact, consent was obtained by the study nurse and the IRB was not informed. Many other important items were not reviewed by the IRB before commencement of the study (e.g. identity of others present during the obtaining of consent; primary care physician to be informed of study participation; insurance for protection of subject; sample CRF including other data collection forms such as diary cards; assurance of the quality or stability of the study medication; current national regulatory authority approval/review or notification; suitability of the study facilities; delegation of responsibility by investigators; the number of study subjects to be included at each site; the means of recruitment of study subjects, such as advertising; and the review decision of other IRBs at other study sites. The IRB was also never notified of a SAE which occurred during the study.

The membership list provided by the IRB did not provide enough information to allow confirmation of some important membership requirements (e.g. members concerned with local issues; no voting member with conflicting interest; at least one experienced clinical investigator; and access to advice from a statistician).

Informed Consent Procedures: There were several irregularities in the consent procedure. Only site personnel (not physicians) informed the study subjects. Discussion with the site personnel and review of the signatures on the consent forms indicated that the persons who obtained consent and informed the study subjects were not medically qualified. The subjects usually did not meet with the investigator or any other physician before agreeing to enter the study. There was no documented evidence that subjects were given sufficient time to consider participation in the study. (Subjects signed consent forms on the same day that they entered the study.) The site personnel indicated that information was provided by telephone before the subjects arrived at the clinic, but this was not adequately documented. Some pages of the consent form were not initialled by some subjects, as required. It seemed that some dates on the consent forms were not personally recorded by the subjects. Twelve consent forms had not been signed by the investigator. Although all other consent forms were signed by the investigator, the study nurse reported that the investigator did not usually see patients before entry to the study. He was asked to sign consent forms later. The obtaining of consent was not documented for 10 subjects by the signature of the authorised investigator (who also signed the study protocol). For eight subjects, a study site co-ordinator had signed in the place of the investigator. For two subjects, there was no signature. All consent forms were also signed by the person obtaining consent: this person was not an authorised investigator. The obtaining of consent was not witnessed for any subjects.

There were some discrepancies between safety information in the information sheet provided to study subjects and information in the investigator brochure. Several items were noted in the information sheet (e.g. chest discomfort, vomiting, lightheadedness, sleeplessness, abdominal pain, rash) which were not included in the investigator brochure.

Protocol: The protocol was signed only by Dr X. At least one other physician (declared on the FDA 1572) was also undertaking investigator responsibilities. Details of the investigators were not provided in the protocol and no list of participating investigators was attached to the protocol.

Several items were missing from the protocol: proposed start and finish date, and duration, of the study; total number of study subjects to be studied at each study site; total number of evaluable subjects required at each study site; means of recruitment of study subjects; source of subjects; definition, policy on replacement and required follow-up for withdrawals/dropouts; procedures for delegation responsibilities; storage conditions for the study medications (the protocol only described storage at 'room temperature', but did not specify acceptable limits of temperature); instructions for safe handling of the study medications; management of clinically significant abnormal clinical laboratory values; procedures for opening individual randomisation codebreak envelopes and revealing the entire randomisation code at the completion of the study; procedures for providing identification of treatment allocation to the investigator at the completion of the study; monitoring frequency; responsibility for preparation of CRFs; instructions for transmittal of CRFs to the sponsor (including method and timeliness); responsibility and timing for data processing and statistical analysis; study subject's primary care physician to be notified of study participation; final clinical report policy; and archiving requirements.

A covering letter for the protocol amendment (issued by the CRO) stated that the protocol change was not a formal amendment, but was an 'administrative change', and therefore did not need approval by the IRB. However, the amendment added an exclusion criterion to the study and added an additional laboratory test and therefore was much more consequential than an 'administrative change'.

CRF Design: Details of the extent of information to be collected in the CRF concerning presenting signs and symptoms, medical history, study medication administration, previous and concomitant medications and AEs were not specified in the protocol. Some discrepancies were noted between the diary card and the protocol concerning the efficacy assessments. The CRF was not modified to reflect the protocol amendment.

Setting Up the Study: There were some discrepancies between safety information in the information sheet provided to study subjects and information in the investigator brochure. Some other important information, particularly relating to management of the study medication, was not included in the investigator brochure. No information about the constituents of the placebo formulation was provided.

The investigator was apparently involved in several other studies (at the time of the audit), although the pre-study report indicated that there were 'no competing studies'. The investigator's personal involvement was apparently limited due to other commitments. At the CRO audit, it was noted that the investigator had conducted 25 studies in the previous two years. The monitor had also indicated concern (in writing) that he was conducting several concurrent studies.

Some important items were not addressed in the pre-study report (e.g. competition with other, similar, studies requiring similar subjects; evidence of retrospective data to support proposed recruitment rate; and availability of environmentally appropriate medication storage facilities). There was no documentation of a formal assessment of the central clinical laboratory prior to use.

Some important information was missing from the initiation reports (e.g. management of biological samples, if any; management (safekeeping and storage) of study medication; management of CRFs including diary cards; information required in the source documents; and procedures for breaking the randomisation code). CRFs, diary cards, and study medication and randomisation code envelopes were not available at the time of the initiation visit. Thus the monitor could not confirm that the supplies arrived safely and were stored properly, and could not demonstrate proper use of the supplies at the initiation visit before treatment of subjects began.

Monitoring: Given the high rate of enrolment and the number of problems detected during the audit, the monitoring frequency was not adequate. Some important items were not documented in the monitor reports (e.g. detailed documentation of source data verification; compliance with inclusion/exclusion criteria, visits required by protocol, concomitant medication use, and procedures; method and timeliness of transmittal of CRFs from investigator site to CRO; number of CRFs transmitted to sponsor; for study medications, check of expiry or 'use before' dates, storage conditions, count/measure of returned medication from subjects to investigator, and correct sequence of allocation of treatment; review of laboratory reference ranges; and biological samples collected, stored, labelled, and transported properly.

Control of Clinical Study Medication: There was no documentation of storage conditions during shipment to the study site. The shipment note did not provide information on handling instructions, storage instructions, quantity, and expiry (or 'use before') date. At the study site, the temperature list was not up to date. A current inventory of study medication was not maintained. The study medication for this study was stored with medications for other studies which were easily observed by the auditors.

Filing/Archiving: The security and indexing of files at the CRO site was confusing. Some records requested of the CRO were dispersed in different locations. Documents from other studies and companies were observed in the same location and were easily accessible. Fire protection involved the use of sprinklers.

Some important documents were missing from both CRO and investigator files. No correspondence with the sponsor/CRO medical adviser with regard to eligibility, evaluability and safety issues noted in the CRFs were observed in the files.

Randomisation codebreak envelopes were not present at the CRO site. There seemed to be some confusion about the requirements for retention of codebreak envelopes. The manufacturing office reported that it had three copies, but was not sure why. The protocol stated that the CRO would have envelopes accessible to the medical monitor, but there was no evidence of compliance with this requirement.

The laboratory protocol indicated that laboratory reports would be delivered overnight to the CRO: none were observed during the audit. CRO personnel stated that reports were being transferred electronically and were all reviewed by the medical monitor: there was no documentation of compliance with these procedures. The laboratory protocol also indicated that weekly status reports would be issued to the CRO, summarising the number of patients tested to date by visit to each investigator site: these summaries were not observed by the auditors.

Source Data: Photocopies of CRFs were used as source documents at the study site. Worksheets (prepared by the CRO) were also used extensively, and were intended to be used as source documents. There were few 'real' source documents which were directly generated by the study site.

The source documents did not provide adequate evidence that subjects met the selection criteria specified by the protocol. The patients were usually recruited by advertisement (newspaper and radio) and many subjects were new to the investigator. Subjects' personal physicians or other physicians knowledgeable about the subjects should have been contacted to provide evidence confirming the subjects' medical history, but there was no evidence that primary care physicians were notified of study participation.

Baseline physical examination, medical history and diagnosis of headache were often not undertaken by the investigator or any other physician. These procedures were usually conducted by a study site co-ordinator. All information about prior headache history was apparently obtained by interview and depended solely on the statements of the study subjects.

There were some discrepancies in data in the subject's clinical record and diary cards compared to data in the CRFs. There were inaccuracies in reporting of AEs. Some reported CRF data were not adequately explained. Examples of discrepancies included:

Subject x: The termination visit physical examination was not done by the investigator or any other physician. Apparently the subject was not seen by a physician throughout the study. (This apparently applied to most subjects in the study according to reports in conversation with the site personnel.) Moderate 'blurred vision', mild 'pulsation in heart', severe 'sensitive to light', moderate 'light-headed', severe 'upset stomach', severe 'pounding in head', moderate 'hot/cold sweats', were noted in the diary card on various dates, but none of these events were noted as AEs in the CRF. The site co-ordinator recorded that these events were 'not new, had before study': however, they were not reported at baseline.

Subject x: 'Worsening of headache' was noted on the AE page. The auditors felt this was inconsistent as it could have applied to many other subjects as well. The patient reported 'sore foot' in the diary card: this was not recorded in the CRF.

Subject x: The CRF page for diary card review indicated that two headaches were treated with study medication. According to the diary card, only one headache was treated. The CRF page for diary card review at the termination visit indicated that three headaches were treated with study medication. According to the diary card, only two headaches were treated.

Reasons were not provided for any data changes. Some data changes (in both CRFs and source documents) were made several months after the original entry. Reasons for these changes should have been provided and the auditors queried the source of the new information.

The dates of the investigator signatures on the inclusion and exclusion criteria pages usually postdated the dates that the study medication was used by the subjects. The auditors queried the intention of the signatures – if they were required to confirm eligibility, they should have predated the date of dosing. The dates of signatures on the 'diary card' review page in the CRF usually postdated the date of the visit (recorded on the same page) indicating that they may not have been reviewed before the subject was allowed to continue in the study.

CHAPTER 3
Ethical Considerations

A major point of difference between the principles of GCP and related disciplines such as GLP and GMP is the emphasis on ethical requirements in GCP. This involves the requirement for review and approval of clinical studies by independent ethics committees/IRBs and the necessity to obtain informed consent from prospective study subjects.

All clinical studies require review by an independent ethics committee/IRB, in accordance with the Declaration of Helsinki, before and during the study. The study files, at both sponsor/CRO and investigator sites must include clear documentation of a 'safe' ethics committee/IRB approval. This means that a general letter of approval is not sufficient. The investigator and the sponsor/CRO need to provide evidence of exactly what was reviewed before and during the study, by whom and when. The independence of the committee must be established (in writing) and the working procedures must be documented to determine how the committee operates (sections 3.1 and 3.2).

A critical ethical aspect of clinical research is that subjects may enter a clinical study conducted by the sponsor/CRO only after being properly informed and indicating consent by signing consent forms. Obtaining informed consent is a complex issue. Again, we must consider who does what, when, what sort of information must be provided, and how it will be documented (sections 3.3 and 3.4).

The sponsor/CRO has a choice of where to place a study and has a duty to place studies in safe settings. Part of the selection process for a study site involves confirming that the ethics committee review will be safe and that all study subjects will be properly informed prior to consent to study participation. If the sponsor/CRO cannot obtain documented evidence at a particular study site of all aspects of the ethics committee/IRB review and cannot confirm that all study subjects will provide informed consent, it is not safe to work with that site.

3.1   ETHICS COMMITTEE/IRB REVIEW AND APPROVAL

Before any study subjects are treated in clinical studies, approval from the committee must be obtained and documented in compliance with international guidelines and the local regulations of the country in which the research is conducted. In practice, in our experience, most studies do not begin before the ethics committee/IRB review: however, when the details of the review are examined carefully, it is evident that compliance with the requirements is not easy to achieve.

Clinical studies begin (for the study subjects) whenever any procedure is undertaken by study subjects which they would not normally undergo: ethics committee/IRB review must be sought before these events. Thus, if a study requires screening procedures, washout from normal treatment, and even completion of a questionnaire which poses personal questions, the study begins when those procedures are undertaken. It is a common misconception that studies begin only when study subjects are randomised to treatment.

Normally, the sponsor/CRO will provide all necessary documentation for submission by the investigator to the ethics committee/IRB. It is not usual procedure for the sponsor/CRO to directly submit items to the committee, unless requested to do so by the committee. Whatever the local variations, the sponsor/CRO is responsible for submitting at least the items in Checklist 3.1–1, in the quantity required by the committee. Some committees require other additional items. This is a daunting list of items to submit, and in fact, we have observed few committees which review all items, as noted by our comments in the checklist.

One important finding of non-compliance with early ethics review was noted in a sample of 321 study sites which we audited. Ethics committees/IRBs did not review full protocols at 41% of the sites. The most common situation contributing to non-compliance was submission of an early draft of the protocol (or only a summary of the protocol) to the ethics committee or IRB with no subsequent follow-up to ensure that the committee received the final protocol. The ethics committees/IRBs were likely unaware that the protocol version which the committee reviewed was not the version eventually used for the study. Many committees only require submission of a completed questionnaire which poses various questions about the study, supplemented by a summary of the protocol. The final protocol may or may not have been submitted with the summary, and it was not clear in the documentation that a protocol was ever submitted in many cases. There were problems with many of these questionnaires which did not always ask the right questions about the study and often seemed to be more concerned about the economics of the study (e.g. costs of overheads) than the safety of the study subjects. Questionnaires or summaries were usually completed by the investigator or sponsor/CRO and thus could have been biased. The design of the questionnaire may also bias the review because it may fail to collect relevant ethical information.

... A study of back pain, UK, 25 patients
The ethics committee agreed to 12 patients: 25 were enrolled at the time of the audit and more were planned. The ethics committee was not informed. This is a very common occurrence. Sponsors/CROs make many changes with regard to numbers of sites, numbers of investigators and numbers of study subjects without informing ethics committees/IRBs. In fact, many ethics committees/IRBs are interested in such changes.

... A study of Alzheimer's disease, Canada, 34 patients
The local ethics committee was more concerned about the use of a

commercial laboratory, instead of the institute's own laboratory, than any other issue. Additionally, screening procedures – drawing blood and withdrawing from normal treatment – were begun before ethics committee approval, before consent and before CRFs arrived at the study site.

. . . A study of hypertension, UK, two sites, 61 patients
Drug supplies were sent to the study sites before ethics committee approval.

. . . A study of allergies, Germany, two sites, 60 patients
All patients were enrolled before ethics committee approval.

. . . A study of stroke, Finland, 600 patients
The ethics committee approved the study in 1986. The protocol was not finalised until 1988.

Prior to selection of a clinical study site, the sponsor/CRO must confirm and document in the pre-study assessment visit report that the investigator has access to a local ethics committee/IRB. Local committees cannot be bypassed: the only exception to this requirement is in France where, by regulation, a central committee may rule for all sites in a multicentre study. If a local ethics committee/IRB is not available, approval to conduct the study should be obtained from the nearest ethic committee/IRB in the country in which the study is being conducted. The selected ethics committees/IRBs should be informed in writing of the reasons for not obtaining local ethic committee/IRB approval. Sponsors/CROs should not conduct studies at sites where the ethics committee/IRB approval is obtained from an ethics committee/IRB in a different country to that in which the study is being conducted. (For example, an ethics committee/IRB ruling for a site in Poland cannot be accepted as the ethics committee/IRB ruling for a site in the UK.)

. . . A study of hypertension, UK , 21 patients
The central ethics committee which had approved the study had been disbanded while the study was ongoing. No local committee was approached, and thus no ethics committee was overseeing the study.

... A study of hypertension, Belgium, 20 patients
Approval by an ethics committee in the UK was accepted by the inves-
tigator and the sponsor/CRO for approval for a site in Belgium. No
local review was sought. The date of approval by the UK committee
postdated the entry of the first study subject in Belgium. The investi-
gator did not have a copy of the approval letter in the study site files.

Sponsors/CROs should generally avoid use of a 'commercial' or 'for profit' or 'for rent' ethics committee/IRB. Obviously the independence and potential conflicts of interest of such committees could be questioned. However, if no other options are available and a 'commercial' ethics committee/IRB must be used, the sponsor/CRO must follow all usual procedures and must be extra diligent to determine that there is no conflict of interest in the selected committee. This is an extraordinary procedure which should be documented, explained and authorised by senior personnel in the sponsor/CRO organisation prior to enrolling subjects at the study site. Sponsor/CROs must not be seen to be 'shopping' for committees of 'convenience' where they know they will receive an uncritical favourable response regardless of the ethical issues.

In any study (single-centre or multicentre), if a local ethics committee/IRB disapproves of a study, the study may not commence at that study site. In multicentre studies, if one local ethics committee/IRB disapproves of a clinical study at a particular study site, all other committees should be notified of this event by the sponsor/CRO, through the investigators. Similarly, the disapproving committee should be notified of approval by other committees. Depending on local regulations, it may also be necessary to notify the national regulatory authorities of disapproval by ethics committees. The sponsor/CRO will always require the investigator to request a written explanation for disapproval from the disapproving committee.

... A study of an anxiolytic, UK, several study sites
The investigator opted for the central 'commercial' ethics committee
because he felt sure the local ethics committee would not approve of the
study (as he reported himself in correspondence with the sponsor/CRO).
One investigator at another site in the UK opted for central committee
review in spite of the request of the local committee to review the study.

At another site, the local ethics committee had disapproved the study because the committee was unhappy with the fact that the study was being conducted by a general practitioner and because patients were being treated with placebo. No attempt by the sponsor/CRO was made to inform other committees of this opinion and the investigator opted for the central committee and disregarded the local committee. The central committee did not inquire about the names of investigators and location of study sites or about local committee review.

... A study of back pain, UK, more than 30 sites
The CRO organised a central ethics committee which approved the study for several study sites. Local committees were not informed, even though it is a requirement in the UK to seek local approval. The central committee did not know or inquire about the names of some of the investigators or the location of study sites.

In many cases it may be necessary to submit documentation to more than one ethics committee/IRB for a single study site. This might occur, for example, if there is a university committee and a hospital committee, or a 'pharmacy' committee and a 'therapeutics' committee which have slightly different interests. All normal procedures should also apply to these other ethics committees/IRBs; however, the sponsor/CRO must ensure that at least one of these committees will provide a review of the ethics of the study.

Proposals for changes and any other recommendations made by the ethics committees/IRB must be considered by the investigator and the sponsor/CRO. The study may not continue at the proposed study site until all such requests have been addressed and any action taken or proposed is communicated to the committee.

... A study of hypertension, Germany, 32 patients
The ethics committee requested close supervision and extra blood pressure measurements to be performed in patients at risk of a rebound phenomenon. No action was taken on this request. The committees rarely check on compliance with their requests – mostly because of lack of resources.

... A study of an anticoagulant, Australia, 26 patients
The ethics committee requested that extra liver function tests be carried out at specific intervals in the study. No action was taken on this request.

... A Phase I study, UK, 17 healthy volunteers
The ethics committee requested a change in the consent form to tell volunteers that they would be receiving placebo. The form was never changed.

... A study of asthma, UK, 10 patients
Patients were not informed that the study was double-blind and that there was a placebo control – the ethics committee approved the incorrect information sheet and consent form. The ethics committee was informed that subjects would receive minor compensation for travel: they received £300.00 each which was described as a 'generous travel allowance'.

Ethics committees/IRBs also have a great responsibility for review during and after clinical studies (Checklist 3.1–2). In other words, committee review is an ongoing responsibility which extends beyond the initial submission of documents to proceed with the study. Many investigators and sponsors/ CROs neglect this duty: the initial review and approval letter is filed away and there is no subsequent correspondence with the committee. Similarly, many ethics committees/IRBs do not ask for any follow-up information on clinical studies. In our audit database of 321 study sites, we were particularly concerned to note that ethics committees were not informed of protocol amendments at 39% of study sites, and at 69% of study sites they were not informed of serious adverse events which occurred during the study. The poor level of compliance is a serious problem internationally especially as the universally stated purpose of ethics committees is to continually assess the risk of the study in the interests of the study subjects. In many cases, local ethics committees/IRBs were not even informed of safety events that occurred in the population for which they had given approval to conduct the study.

Given the workload of most committees, the fact that they are voluntary unpaid organisations in many countries, and the finding that they are often unaware of GCP requirements, it is not surprising that there is much non-compliance with regard to the ethics committee/IRB review. However, the sponsor/CRO must nevertheless undertake careful management of the ethical review to assure compliance to the highest standards possible. Some regulators, particularly the FDA, will reject submissions if they are not satisfied with the ethics committee/IRB review.

Checklist 3.1–1. Review by Ethics Committees/IRBs Before Clinical Studies Begin

Ethics committees/IRBs must review the following items before clinical studies are allowed to proceed:

- Protocol (full): the submitted protocol must have previously received the signed approval of investigators and the sponsor/CRO. A summary of the protocol may also be requested by some committees and the investigator may request the sponsor/CRO to assist in preparing the summary. The summary cannot substitute for the full protocol, although it is not necessary for each member of the committee to review the full protocol.
- Sample CRFs and other data collection forms (e.g. diary cards and quality of life forms): all proposed data collection forms should be appended to the protocol. Committees rarely ask for this document although it is supposed to be an annex to the protocol: thus, the committee does not review and confirm the planned data capture which is usually inadequately described in the protocol.
- Consent procedures (described in the protocol and the appended information sheet and consent form) which specify who will be obtaining consent, how consent will be documented and whether or not a witness will be present;
- Identity of persons who will provide information and seek consent: committees are usually not informed that the declared investigators might not be the actual persons obtaining consent.
- Consent form/information sheet: most committees will be particularly interested in these documents to ensure that all necessary information is provided to study subjects.
- Suitability of investigator and facilities, including support personnel: some committees may request a copy of investigator and other site personnel CVs. The committee will be particularly interested in allo-

cation of resources, whether the investigator has enough time and patients to conduct the study, and whether use of resources for clinical studies will detract from normal medical care requirements. (In a multicentre study, identification of other investigators and locations should be provided to each local committee.)

- Delegation of responsibility by investigators: committees are rarely informed that patients may not actually be seen by the physicians who signed the protocol.
- Source of study subjects and means of recruitment: the committee will wish to know if study subjects are known to investigators and if not (i.e. referred patients), how investigators will confirm eligibility and whether primary care practitioners will be informed.
- Appropriateness (eligibility) of study subjects (described in the protocol);
- Primary care physician to be informed of study participation;
- Means of recruitment of study subjects (e.g. advertising);
- Text of advertisements, if any, for recruitment of study subjects: the committee will wish to determine that advertisements are not unduly coercive or misleading or too 'inviting'.
- Number of subjects to be studied and justification for sample size. (This information should be in the protocol.) The committee will be interested in how many subjects will be exposed to the risk of treatment. In a multicentre study, the local ethics committee/IRB should be informed of the number of subjects to be enrolled at each site and the total number of subjects to be enrolled in the study.
- Investigator brochure or other authorised summary of information (e.g. preclinical and clinical summaries) about the investigational products, including comparator products and placebo: if the study medication/device is a marketed product, the ethics committee/IRB must review the most current data sheet, product monograph, etc. The brochure is particularly important for confirming the formal declared safety profile of the study treatment and therefore is of great assistance to committees in assessing the relevance of AEs. Also, the committee can verify, by reviewing the brochure or product labelling, that the information sheet for obtaining consent provided sufficient information with regard to safety.
- Evidence of regulatory submission and review/approval (if applicable): committees particularly wish to know whether the drug/device is on the market in their country or in other countries, and the details of the stage of the submission.

- Adequacy of confidentiality safeguards, with regard to protection of identification of the study subject (described in the protocol and the appended information sheet and consent form);
- Insurance provisions, if any, for injury to study subjects (described in the protocol or provided as a separate document). Committees must confirm that there is insurance for protection of the study subjects – which is different from indemnity or insurance for other parties. Committees make many assumptions about insurance, often misunderstanding that indemnity for the investigator or the institution does not necessarily protect the study subject.
- Compensation/treatment for injury to study subjects;
- Indemnity/insurance provisions for the sponsor/CRO, investigator, institution, etc. (as relevant to the study and if required by local regulations).
- Payments or rewards to be made to study subjects, if any: committees must determine that the amount, and schedule of payments, is not unduly coercive.
- Benefits, if any, to study subjects;
- Payments or rewards to be made to investigators: review of this item is changing dramatically because of the increasing interest in the potential conflict of interest for the investigator if he/she benefits materially from the study. Ten years ago this item was rarely considered; now we observe more and more committees asking questions. Many committees are beginning to realise that the financial interests of the investigator might have a strong influence on some aspects of the study, particularly recruitment patterns.
- Assurance of quality/stability of medication/device to be administered: this should be of interest to the committee, to ensure that the product is safe, but it is rarely considered.
- Review decision of other ethics committees/IRBs in multicentre studies: usually committees are not even informed of disapproval or restrictions on approval by other committees.
- Duration of study;
- Plans to review data collected to ensure safety.

Checklist 3.1–2. Review by Ethics Committees/IRBs During and After Clinical Studies

During and after clinical studies, ethics committees/IRBs should review the following items:

- Serious and/or unexpected AEs, if any occur during the study, including the follow-up period: if a study is expected to involve many SAEs (e.g. studies in advanced stages of cancer), it may be necessary to negotiate with the ethics committee/IRB to determine specifically which types of SAEs the committee should be notified of immediately and if a reasonable time period (e.g. every three months) for reporting summaries of SAEs would be acceptable. All safety information which is considered important enough to be reported to regulatory authorities should also be reported to the local committee.
- Protocol amendments, if any;
- Reasons for protocol amendments;
- Protocol violations which impact on subject safety, if any;
- Discontinuation of study, if applicable and any reasons for premature discontinuation;
- Any new significant information (e.g. information arising from other studies, results of interim analyses, marketing approvals, changes in local procedures, updated investigator brochure, supply problems) during study, if any;
- Amendments to consent form/information sheet, if any;
- Annual reports of the study: the ethics committees/IRB should review the progress of a clinical study at least once each year. More frequent review may be necessary, depending on the working procedures of each individual ethics committee.
- Final clinical report/summary of study: it is not normal procedure to submit the full report in the format prepared for a regulatory submission: an abbreviated version is more appropriate for the ethics committee/IRB.
- Publications, if any.

3.2 DOCUMENTATION OF SAFE ETHICS COMMITTEE/IRB APPROVAL

To document safe ethics committee/IRB review and approval, the sponsor/CRO and the investigator must retain (in their respective archives) evidence of all correspondence, review and approval letters, committee membership lists and written committee working procedures.

The ethics committee/IRB review and/or approval letter and/

or statement to conduct a clinical study should clearly indicate the items in Checklist 3.2–1. In practice, few committees will provide this amount of detailed information and so some 'upward management' may be necessary. (Our audit database of 321 sites showed that review letters did not adequately indicate the following items: list of items reviewed (65% non-compliance), list of members attending review meetings (64%); and specific identification of protocol version (61%).) A wise sponsor/CRO will submit the documentation with a covering letter which specifies exactly what was submitted and prompts the committee to indicate approval on the covering letter or another form. Most committees are agreeable to such a procedure. However, if the committee offers some resistance, it should be firmly stated that the sponsor/CRO must have the relevant information to survive possible future inspections. (This applies also to the documentation of committee membership and working procedures as discussed below.)

. . . A study of hormone replacement therapy, UK, 35 study subjects
The title of the study on the ethics committee approval letter indicated that a double-blind study would be conducted. In fact, the final protocol referred to a single-blind study. This occurred because an early draft of the protocol was submitted to the committee and the pharmaceutical company later discovered that it could not prepare double-blind medications. The committee was not informed.

The membership of an ethics committee/IRB will vary nationally and regionally. However, the sponsor/CRO is only permitted to conduct studies that are approved by ethics committees/IRBs which have a sufficient number of qualified members to enable a medical and scientific review of the proposed study and to enable a review of all other ethical aspects of the study (Checklist 3.2–1). Details of the membership of the ethics committee/IRB should be obtained and reviewed by the sponsor/CRO, prior to initiating the study, to ascertain the above and to determine that there is no serious conflict of interest (e.g. investigator voting on her/his study). If there is a conflict of interest, there must be written evidence that the committee member with the conflict of interest did not participate in the voting or decision-making procedure. Invited ad hoc members also may not vote (depending on the working procedures of the committee) and must be identified. If the ethics committee/IRB regularly reviews studies involving vulnerable populations (e.g. children, elderly, unconscious, mentally impaired, students, employees, etc.), at least one member should primarily be concerned with the welfare of those potential study subjects. If there is difficulty in any of these areas, the sponsor must query the situation carefully or declare the study site as ineligible.

The issue of conflict of interest must be particularly carefully addressed as our audit findings indicate that the ethics committee/IRB included a member with a potential serious conflict of interest (e.g. an investigator) or the ethics committee/IRB membership list did not provide adequate information to assess the potential conflict of interest at 56% of 378 sites. The poor level of compliance with this item was mostly due to lack of evidence to assess potential conflict of interest. This finding was probably due to individual sponsor/CRO procedures: the requirement to assess ethics committee membership list for potential conflicts of interest was rarely addressed in SOPs and it did not seem that sponsors/CROs took this item seriously. In those cases where investigators were discovered by the auditors to be members of the ethics committee, there was no clear documentation to indicate that the investigator had withdrawn from the decision-making process of the ethics committee.

Membership lists must be dated, current (not more than one year old) and must identify the relevant institution/authority.

... A study of alcohol dependence, Germany, 26 patients
The investigator's 'boss' had financial interests in the study and chaired the ethics committee.

... A phase I study, Canada, 12 healthy volunteers
The secretary of the ethics committee (established by a CRO) was also the CRO's quality assurance manager.

... Studies in psychotropic drugs, USA
The chairperson of the IRB was also responsible for a multi-million dollar research budget at the large teaching hospital where he was employed.

. . . A study of cardiovascular surgery, Germany, 21 patients
The anaesthetist for the study was on the ethics committee and person-
ally voted to approve the protocol. He was also listed as an investigator
and every patient at this site was administered a prohibited (by
protocol) anaesthetic agent by this same anaesthetist: the patients
were all declared ineligible in the final analysis. Many researchers
do not appreciate the serious effect of such protocol violations
on the final analysis. A study begins with a statistically determined sample size such that the minimum number of patients
possible are exposed to the risk of the study while still allowing
for a reasonable statistical analysis. Each study subject that is lost
for the analysis because of protocol violations diminishes the
sample size. This particular multicentre study was eventually
abandoned because there were too few patients for the final
analysis. In effect, more than 500 patients were treated to no
useful purpose.

. . . A study of diabetes, Canada, 22 patients
The ethics committee membership consisted of two 'Drs' and two
'professors'. The sponsor could not find a copy of the ethics committee
approval letter. Many ethics committees are 'stacked' with physicians – some have no lay people at all – in spite of universally
stated requirements that ethics committees/IRBs should not
consist of only medical personnel.

. . . A study of an anxiolytic, Germany, nine patients
The ethics committee consisted of one person. (The CRO was having
difficulty obtaining a list of ethics committee members. The auditors
determined from the investigator that the chairperson of the local
'chamber of physicians' had assumed the role of ethics committee.
There was no membership list because there was no ethics committee!)

The sponsor/CRO should request a copy of the working procedures of the ethics committee/IRB (Checklist 3.2–3). The
working procedures should be dated and current, and should
identify the specific committee/IRB. If the monitor is unable to
obtain the working procedures, the reason must be documented
and there should be a note in the file to explain why a decision
was made to proceed at this study site. If any serious irregularities are noted, the sponsor/CRO should determine whether or

not it is safe to proceed with the study at the intended study site. A detailed set of working procedures should provide sufficient information to assure sponsors/CROs, investigators, auditors and inspectors of the integrity of the ethics committee/IRB. Unfortunately, today, it is still difficult to obtain working procedures from many committees.

Like membership lists, working procedures must be dated, current (not more than one year old) and must identify the relevant institution/authority.

Checklist 3.2–1. Documentation of Ethics Committees/IRB Review and Approval

The ethics committee/IRB review or approval letter should specify the following items:
- Date of review/approval;
- Date of review/approval meeting and indication of a meeting;
- Specific identification of protocol version (e.g. draft number or 'final' or date). (Non-specification accounts for why many committees were not aware of which version was approved.)
- Identification of the protocol by the correct title. (Sometimes the title was changed by the committee.)
- List of items reviewed: this list may be ascertained by review of the submission to the ethics committee/IRB;
- List of members who attended meeting (and list of members who voted on whether or not to approve the study);
- Any conditions for approval and means of satisfying those conditions.

Checklist 3.2–2. Membership of Ethics Committees/IRBs*

The ethics committee/IRB membership should comprise at least the following:

---

* This list is compiled from several guidelines and regulations. Not all items are required in all countries: however, most of them would be considered as good practice in all countries. The reader is advised to check on specific national requirements.

- At least five members and not more than 15–18 members;
- Sufficiently qualified (to assess research) members. (Not every member needs to be an expert, but at least one must have expertise in clinical research.)
- Members concerned with local issues;
- Individuals not entirely of one profession;
- No (voting) member with conflicting interest and at least one member with no relationship to the institution in which research is conducted. (This is a particular requirement of the FDA to assure independence as, by definition, Institutional Review Boards (IRBs) may only comprise members belonging to the institution.)
- At least one medically qualified member and at least one non-medically qualified member;
- At least one non-scientific member (lay person) and at least one experienced clinical investigator;
- At least one general practitioner (this is a particular requirement in those countries in which patients are registered with general practitioners or family doctors, e.g. UK, Canada) and at least one nurse. (The Royal College of Physicians of London specifies a nurse in 'active practice' with patients.)
- Access to advice from at least one pharmacist – some countries require pharmacists as permanent members, e.g. France, a biostatistician, and a legally qualified person (e.g. a lawyer). (Some countries require lawyers as permanent members, e.g. Germany.)
- At least one member of each sex.

Checklist 3.2–3. Working Procedures of Ethics Committees/IRBs*

The working procedures of ethics committees/IRBs should indicate compliance with the following policies:
- Items to be reviewed were specified;
- Membership requirements were specified;
- Frequency of meetings was specified;

---

* This list is compiled from several guidelines and regulations. Not all items are required in all countries: however, most of them would be considered as good practice in all countries. The reader is advised to check on specific national requirements.

- Decision-making procedures (e.g. voting quorum, majority vote, chairperson action) were specified, and the investigator was to be excluded from vote;
- No significant changes in studies were to be permitted without ethics committee/IRB approval, and prompt reporting by the investigator of new risks (arising during the study) to study subjects was required;
- Procedures for suspension, termination or withdrawal of approval were defined, authority to intervene was defined, and procedures for disciplining non-compliant investigators was defined;
- Communication with other ethics committees/IRBs was required in multicentre studies;
- Maintenance of confidentiality of sponsor/CRO information was required;
- Review of studies was required to be conducted at least annually;
- Copies of correspondence were required to be maintained and minutes of meetings were required to be recorded. Records were required to be maintained for a specified period (e.g. at least three years).
- Receipt of the final clinical study report from the sponsor/CRO was required, and receipt of publications from the sponsor/CRO was required.

3.3   CONDUCT OF INFORMED CONSENT

A subject may enter a clinical study conducted by the sponsor/ CRO only after he/she has been properly informed and has signed a consent form. The general principles for the conduct of informed consent are noted in Checklist 3.3–1. Our finding is that most study sites comply with this basic requirement, but there were some significant problems with the consent procedure, in examples as noted below, which might lead some reviewers to consider that safe informed consent was not obtained in many cases.

Under normal circumstances a clinical study should not be conducted unless informed consent can be obtained from either the study subjects or authorised legal representatives. The normal procedure for obtaining informed consent may only be circumvented if the investigator and a second physician not otherwise participating in the study certify all the following, in writing: a life-threatening situation confronts the subject and necessitates use of the study medication/device; informed consent cannot be obtained because of the inability to communicate with or obtain legally effective informed consent from the subject; there is insufficient time to obtain consent from the subject's legal representative; and there is no alternative method of approved or generally recognised therapy which would provide an equal or greater likelihood of saving the subject's life.

The ethics committee/IRB must be advised of all the procedures to be followed in the process of obtaining informed consent prior to subject enrolment and of any deviation from these procedures during the conduct of a clinical study.

Our review of 328 study sites indicated that informed consent was not obtained before the start of the study at 38% of sites. At many sites there was simply not a good understanding of when a study actually began. Further, the documentation did not indicate that consent was obtained from qualified investigators at 48% of study sites. The poorest level of compliance for this item is in the USA and the UK, where there is much reliance on 'study co-ordinators', who basically take over the study at many investigator sites. The amount of delegation in these countries was such that the auditors have observed many situations where study subjects were never seen by designated investigators (and sometimes never seen by a physician!). In France and Germany where the level of compliance for this item is better, physicians were much more directly connected to their study subjects and did not delegate so easily. Or, if there was delegation, it was much more likely to be to another physician. Sponsor/CRO standards also contribute to this problem by not clearly specifying the criteria for qualified investigators and investigator responsibilities.

... A study of cardiovascular surgery, UK, six patients
The consent dates, originally dated after the start of the study, were changed (by overwriting) to indicate that the patient had provided consent before the study started.

... A study of thrombosis, UK, 68 patients
Seventeen different physicians had signed the consent forms: the forms

were subsequently countersigned by one of the two authorised investigators two to four weeks after consent was obtained. This is a common finding indicating the absence of the investigator at the time consent was obtained. What is the purpose of the countersignatures?

... A study of cardiovascular surgery, France, 28 patients
There was no place to record the date of consent on the consent form.

... A study of hypertension, Canada, 15 patients
The investigator signed consent forms up to two months after the forms were signed by the patients. The study nurse reported that she was the only person involved in the consent process and she left the forms on his desk for signature at some later date. Again, what was the purpose of the investigator signatures?

... A study of coronary artery disease, Northern Ireland, 16 patients
All subjects had also signed a consent form (observed in the file by the auditors) for another concurrent study using an unlicensed imaging agent to measure ejection fractions. Several patients had started on this other study, but nothing was reported in the CRFs. Patients can only take part in one study at a time!

... A study of cardiovascular surgery, UK, seven patients
The sponsor designed a consent form which only provided space for the names and signatures of the study subject and a witness. There was no witness to the study. The investigator signed as the witness!

... A study of cardiovascular surgery, several sites in Europe
The sponsor designed a consent form which did not have space to record the date of the patient's consent. Several hundred patients had signed the forms by the time the audits were undertaken.

... A Phase I study in healthy sterilised female volunteers, UK, 20 volunteers
The consent form required the signature of a company (sponsor) representative. These individuals were not present when consent was obtained. What was the purpose of this signature? Is there a breach of confidentiality, or a conflict of interest, if sponsor/ CRO personnel are present during the consent procedure?

... A study of coronary artery disease, UK, 25 patients
The investigator signed the consent forms as both the 'informer' and the 'witness.'. The sponsor retained the consent forms in their archives with patient names clearly identifiable.

... A study of back pain, UK, 25 patients
The investigator signed the consent form as the witness. The ethics committee had requested, and had been assured, that the consent process would be independently witnessed.

... A study of cardiovascular surgery, USA, 28 patients
Consent forms for 'other' studies, signed but not dated by study subjects in the current study, were noted in the medical files. Several of these forms were not dated or signed by investigators or the investigator signature postdated the subject signatures. The auditors could not tell from review of the source documents whether or not these other studies were being conducted.

... A Phase I study, UK, 17 healthy volunteers
Eleven forms were signed by unidentifiable 'investigators'. This is a common finding. A physician, who happened to be on duty at the time the study subject was approached for study participation, was involved in the obtaining of consent. He or she had not signed the protocol and there was no evidence that they were qualified to obtain consent.

... A study of hormone replacement therapy, France, 19 study subjects
There were several consent problems: three study subjects did not consent; four subjects did not date the consent forms, nine subjects signed on a different day from that of the investigator and 11 subjects did not consent before treatment.

... A study of prostate cancer, UK, 32 patients
The study site co-ordinator signed in place of the investigator for all patients. This common occurrence is usually indicative of problems in defining investigator responsibilities and appropriately delegating tasks.

... A study of prostate cancer, UK, 24 patients
Signed consent forms were missing for 17 subjects. With such a high

proportion of missing forms, the auditors and inspectors might well suspect that consent was never obtained!

... A study of diabetes, Canada, 21 patients
The investigator countersigned the consent forms after the patient was entered into the study. Consent was actually obtained by the study site co-ordinator.

Checklist 3.3–1. Principles for the Conduct of Informed Consent

The following principles for conducting informed consent must be adhered to in all clinical studies:

- Informed consent must be obtained from each study subject. The person receiving the information and giving consent must sign the consent form. This is usually the study subject, but may be the study subject's legally acceptable representative (depending on national regulations) in the event that the study subject is incapable of providing informed consent (e.g. the subject is unable to write or understand the consent documents), or the study subject is in a 'vulnerable' population (e.g. children, elderly). Subjects who cannot understand (read, write or comprehend) the national language may be ineligible for studies which require subjective interpretation (e.g. completion of quality of life forms).
- Informed consent must be obtained before the start of the study;
- The person providing the information and obtaining consent must sign the consent form. This person must be an investigator who must be qualified to adequately inform the study subject and therefore must have signed the protocol to indicate full knowledge of all aspects of the study. His/her signature also indicates personal involvement in the consent process. If other personnel (e.g. study nurse) assist in providing information or obtaining consent, he/she should also sign the consent form, clearly describing their role in the consent procedure. Dates of investigator signatures should precede the start of the study (for the study subject). Investigators and study subjects must personally date their signatures.
- A witness or patient advocate should be present during the consent procedure at the times of providing information and giving consent and must sign the consent form. The witness will ensure that there was no coercion in the obtaining of informed consent and that the

study subject was given adequate time to consider participation in the study. The witness must be able to confirm that the consent procedure was adequate and must have no vested interest in the clinical study (i.e. the witness should be impartial, independent or neutral as far as this can be achieved). The relationship of the witness to the study subject and to the investigator or the study should be documented. The witness should receive an explanation that he/she is a witness to the consent procedure, not only a witness to the signatures on the consent form. The usual policy of the sponsor/CRO should be to require consent to be witnessed in all circumstances. However, if the local circumstances or certain aspects of the study prohibit the use of a witness, this must be explained and documented in writing. In cases in which the ethics committees/IRB requires a witness, but the investigator is reluctant to use a witness, this must be brought to the attention of the ethics committee. The consent form must provide a space for the signature (and date) of a witness. The witness should be independent of the study.

3.4   INFORMATION TO BE PROVIDED TO STUDY SUBJECTS IN CLINICAL STUDIES

The requirements for informed consent will be stated in the protocol and in SOPs. The task of drafting the proposed information sheet and consent form should be undertaken as soon as the protocol is final. (This is usually done initially by the sponsor/CRO.) The investigator should be invited to comment on the proposed information sheet and consent form prior to finalisation, taking into account knowledge of the local ethics committee/IRB requirements. The sponsor/CRO will determine, at the study site assessment visits, whether there are any standardised forms or formats required by specific study sites, which might necessitate further revision of the information sheet and consent form.

All information sheets and consent forms should include the items in Checklist 3.4–1. Before release as an attachment to the final protocol (and therefore, before release to ethics committees/IRBs and regulatory authorities (if applicable), the proposed information sheet and consent form must be reviewed and approved internally by the sponsor/CRO. If further changes are required, subsequent to external review by the ethics committees/IRBs and/or the regulatory authority, the proposed changes must be reviewed and approved prior to the enrolment of study subjects. If an omission or addition is requested by an external reviewer (e.g. ethics committees/IRB or regulatory authority), an explanation must be documented.

If there are any changes to the protocol and/or if significant events (e.g. SAEs) occur during the study, the consent form and information sheet must be reviewed to determine if amendments to them are required. If the consent form and/or information sheet are amended, this information must be submitted to the ethics committee/IRB. It may also be necessary to submit the revised documents to the regulatory authority, if applicable, in the country in which the study is being conducted. Finally, it may also be necessary to reinform study subjects and obtain consent again.

... A study of diabetes, Canada, 21 patients
The patients were not informed that they would only receive placebo for four weeks prior to randomisation.

... A study of dyspepsia, UK, 57 patients
The study subjects were not informed in information sheets or consent forms that they would be subjected to endoscopy, biopsy and ultrasonography during the study. It is easy to overlook the fact that some procedures would not be conducted for normal treatment of the presenting condition, but patients must be informed of treatments which would not usually be undertaken.

... A study of hormone replacement therapy, Canada, 13 study subjects
Patients were not informed that ultrasound tests would be conducted during the study.

... A study of coronary artery disease, UK, 25 patients
With regard to compensation for injury, the protocol referred to German legal requirements. (The head office of the pharmaceutical company was in Germany.) The study subjects were not informed of any local compensation: this was approved by the local UK ethics committee. Few ethics committees/IRBs confirm that compensation offered in another country is applicable to their own

country. Also, the terms of compensation are often not well explained to study subjects.

... A study of an anticoagulant, Italy, 15 patients
Patients in the study were not informed that the study medication had become available on the market during the time of the study. Consequently, patients continued to be treated with placebo when they could have received the marketed product. The investigator was also on the ethics committee and had decided not to inform the committee. If the study medication had been approved for marketing, obviously a decision had been made that it was safe and effective. It was not fair to treat subjects with placebo when a safe treatment was available without informing them of the risk.

... A study of asthma, UK, 10 patients
Patients were not informed that the study was double-blind and that there was a placebo control.

... A study of cancer, UK, four patients
The information sheet did not inform subjects that they would all receive placebo at some stage in the study.

Checklist 3.4–1. Items for Informed Consent

The information sheets and consent forms should contain the following items:

1. Information about the consent procedure:
- Consent to be given by the study subject's free will;
- Adequate time (which must be defined in advance in the protocol) must be allowed for the study subject to decide on participation in the study. He/she must confirm this on the consent form. This is a very tricky issue and most consent forms which we review give us the impression that little or no time was allowed when the dates were compared to the date of study entry. One of the best guidelines we have seen is that of a UK source which states that at least 24 hours must be provided unless there is a good rationale for a shorter time period. (If the study involves acute or emergency presentations, then there might be some justification for a shorter

time period.) The time proposed should be brought to the attention of the local ethics committee.

- Adequate time to ask questions;
- Statement that participation is entirely voluntary;
- Statement that refusal to participate would involve no penalties or loss of usual benefits;
- Description of the circumstances under which participation would be terminated. It might be very important to let the subject know in advance that their participation might be terminated if the treatment does not work so they will not suspect another more sinister reason.
- Right to withdraw at any time without prejudice or consequences;
- Study subject is allowed to keep the written explanation (information sheet and consent form) for future reference.

2. Information about the study and medications/devices:
- Instructions on use and storage of study medication/device, if relevant,
- Name of sponsor/CRO;
- Explanation that the study is a research procedure;
- Description of study type and research aims;
- Description of study medications/devices;
- Description of procedures to be followed;
- Description of experimental procedures to be followed, if any. Experimental procedures might include those which are not normally used for the presentation under consideration or procedures which are new or have never been used before.
- Comparator treatments (including placebo) described: it is important to explain 'placebo' in simple terms.
- Randomisation procedures: randomisation is not easily understood by many subjects and should also be explained in simple terms.
- Expected duration of participation;
- Required number of visits;
- Reason for selection of suitable subjects: an explanation of why the subject had been approached for study participation might give the subject a better understanding of the study.
- Approximate number of other study subjects participating in the study: it might be important for the subject to appreciate that they are one of a thousand others rather than the first person participating in the study.

3. Information about the risks/benefits:

- Foreseeable risks, discomforts, side effects and inconveniences described;
- Known therapeutic benefits, if any, described. The benefits must not be 'oversold'.
- Availability of alternative therapies described. If there are other treatments, this must be explained so that the subject does not feel the new treatment is their only option.
- Any new findings, which might affect the safety of the study subject, and that become available during participation in the study will be disclosed to the study subject;
- Assurance of compensation for treatment-induced injury with specific reference to local guidelines. (It must not be expected that the study subject is familiar with the guidelines and therefore they must be explained and/or attached.)
- Terms of compensation;
- Measures to be taken in the event of an AE or therapeutic failure;
- Financial remuneration, if any: patients, whether receiving therapeutic benefit or not, are not usually paid for participation in clinical research, except for incidentals such as travel costs. Healthy volunteers are usually paid a fee for participation, but this payment should never be offered to induce the prospective subjects to take risks they would not normally take.
- Explanation of additional costs that may result from participation, if any. (This normally occurs only in the USA.)

4. Other items:

- Ethics committee/IRB approval obtained;
- Name of ethics committee/IRB (if applicable by local and/or national requirements), and details of contact person on the ethics committee/IRB (if applicable by local and/or national requirements);
- Explanation that participation is confidential, but records (which divulge study subject names) may be reviewed by authorised representatives of the sponsor/CRO and may be disclosed to a regulatory authority. Study subjects were often not adequately informed (in the information sheet or consent form) that confidential records (i.e. source documents) would be reviewed by the monitor or other sponsor/CRO representatives (e.g. auditors) or the regulatory authority (e.g. inspectors).
- Name, address and telephone number (24-hour availability) of

contact person at study site for information or in the event of an emergency. (This information may be provided on a separate card.)
- Requirement to disclose details of medical history, any medicines (or alcohol) currently being taken, changes in any other medication/ device use and details of participation in other clinical studies;
- Medical records will clearly identify study participation;
- Conditions as they apply to women of child-bearing potential;
- Primary care physician (or general practitioner or family doctor) and/ or referring physician will be informed of study participation and any significant problems arising during the study. Some subjects may not be comfortable with this requirement – for example, in a study of sexually transmitted diseases, they may not wish the doctor, perhaps a family friend, to be aware of their situation. If this is the case, the subject is not eligible for the study as it is vital to confirm history with the primary care physician.
- The information sheet must be written in language which is under-standable (e.g. technically simple and in the appropriate national language) to the study subject.

CASE STUDY THREE

A Comparative Study of Drug X in the Treatment of Malaria in Approximately 200 Adults (Far East).

This study was conducted in the Far East, where there are few formal rules for clinical studies. Which rules would you apply? Can we impose ethical standards on different countries/cultures? Although many readers might have problems with the ethical standard applied, this study had reasonably good standards other-wise, compared to many studies conducted in the 'developed' world.

Summary of Major Deficiencies

Standard Operating Procedures: The CRO did not have SOPs for many important topics including protocols and protocol amendments, CRF design, statistical procedures, randomisation procedures, study medication management, reporting AEs, closure of a clinical study, clinical study reports, filing and archiving of documents, auditing and detection and management of fraud. Insufficient detail was provided on informed consent and data management procedures.

Ethics Committee Review: The ethics committee approval document was not dated and did not contain the correct title for the protocol. (In fact the title referred to approval of 'comparative clinical trials', in the plural!) The investigator obtained the date of approval by telephoning the ethics committee during the audit. The specific protocol used for the study was not submitted to the ethics committee and thus much of the information that the ethics committee should have reviewed was not available. A summary of the protocol was sent to the committee: it appeared that the summary reflected the study, but this could not be verified as the document was not written in English. The ethics committee was not informed of a change in dosing of the study medication. (No protocol amendment was ever prepared for this change.)

Informed Consent Procedures: The information provided in the combined information sheet and consent form was brief and did not include many important items (e.g. the fact that blood would be drawn for purposes of assay levels, approximate number of other study subjects in the study, reasons for selection of subjects, risks, discomforts, availability of alternative therapies, compensation or insurance, contact information, conditions applying to child-bearing women and the fact that new findings were to be disclosed). The information sheet indicated that the subject *might* receive the study medication or the comparative drug and did not adequately explain the probability of the subject receiving one drug or the other. Subjects were required to remain in the hospital for 28 days, but this was not explained.

Because of language problems and illiteracy of the study subjects it was difficult to document informed consent. All study subjects in the sample selected for audit provided written consent to participate in the study by signing the consent form with their initials, name or *thumb print*. The obtaining of consent was not documented for all study subjects by the signature of the investigator. Only the name of the investigator was included in the information sheet. The investigator had not signed the consent form. The dates of consent form signatures preceded the actual study entry for all except eight patients who signed the consent one to six days after enrolment.

Discussion with the investigator suggested that he personally provided information to all study subjects in the presence of a witness, a nurse. (The protocol allowed for consent to be provided by the parent/guardian of the patient, but there was no space on the consent form for this person's signature.) Apparently the information was provided verbally and in writing. However, the subjects were not given a copy of the information sheet because many of them could not read or write.

The original signed consent forms were archived by the CRO, who would thus have confidential patient names in their archives.

Protocol: Significant deficiencies in the protocol were: no indication of labelling requirements (tear-off labels were attached to the CRFs but these did not have all the details on the label stuck to the bottle); no descriptions of the procedures for handling blood samples and the amount of blood for assay of drug levels and parasite sensitivity testing (requirements for storage and processing of plasma samples for measurement of plasma concentrations of study medication were not stated); AEs were only to be recorded during the first seven days of the study period; SAEs were only to be reported immediately if they were considered to be 'possibly or reasonably attributable' to the investigational drug (there was no requirement to immediately report SAEs that were 'not reasonably attributable' to the investigational drug or that occurred in association with the comparative drug); no statements concerning clinically significant abnormal clinical laboratory values being reported as AEs; no requirements for the archiving of documents by the investigator; no indication of the regulatory requirements; and a statement that study subjects were to be compensated for injury in accordance with ABPI guidelines. (What would the Association of British Pharmaceutical Industries (ABPI), mean to investigators and patients in the Far East?)

CRF Design: Some of the data required by the 'admission examination', 'clinical assessments', 'other medications' and 'patient summary record' CRF pages were not described in the protocol. Space was not provided in the CRF to record some of the data required by the protocol (e.g. vital signs and parasitology). Some essential data (e.g. previous and concurrent medical conditions, physical examinations after admission, unexpected AEs and AEs related to abnormal laboratory data, information concerning SAEs) were not required to be recorded by either the protocol or CRF. The protocol required vital signs to be monitored every six hours during the acute stage and blood pressure to be measured at least daily. There was no space in the CRF for recording these data. A copy of the temperature chart which contained much of this information was to be attached to the completed CRF but this did not occur. The 'parasitology' form did not provide space for the required period and for follow-up parasitology.

Setting Up the Study: The investigator brochure (which was actually only a document entitled 'clinical report') was not up to date and did not contain some of the necessary details (e.g. identification and approval of sponsor, summary of possible medication interactions, summary of contraindications and precautions and management of spill or accidental exposure or overdose). Files containing details of the monitoring staffs' training and qualifications were not maintained by the CRO. The investigator's CV did not contain sufficient detail of his qualifications. The study site assessment report had insufficient detail concerning storage of study medication, space, equipment and laboratories. The study site agreements only required the reporting of AEs attributable to the investigational drug.

Monitoring: Monitoring was not conducted frequently, only every three to four months. (The sponsor only required the CRO to conduct four monitoring visits during the study.)

Control of Clinical Study Medication: Shipment documents did not adequately describe the requirements for the environmental conditions, batch numbers and expiry dates for the study medication. The withdrawal of a number of study subjects' medication from within the randomised blocks caused confusion and might have compromised the randomisation process. Some dispensing details were recorded on various scattered documents on the wards, making it difficult to reconcile information.

Filing/Archiving: The investigator archives were not secure: documents were stored in cardboard boxes on the floor in the office of the investigator.

Source Data: As some of the patient records were written in the national language it was not possible to determine whether the study subject initials on the CRFs matched the surnames and forenames on the source medical records for all study subjects in the sample selected for audit. All pages on the CRFs matched those on the source records in the sample selected for audit.

In all study subjects in the sample selected for audit, the source medical records did not clearly indicate (by date, study medication identification and study title) participation in the study. Patients enrolled in the study did not have family doctors and were not apparently referred by other physicians: thus it was not possible to confirm medical history. Patients came to the hospital as a result of 'word-of-mouth' or previous experience.

Details of concurrent medications (including placebo given to patients to satisfy them that they were being adequately treated) were recorded in the source documents. However, some of these medications were not recorded in the CRF. A decision had apparently been made to record and analyse only the concomitant medications for the first seven days of the study.

AEs were not adequately reported in eight study subjects of the sample selected for audit. The CRF was not designed to indicate, and comment upon, clinically significant out-of-range laboratory values. The only data recorded in the CRF were the actual laboratory values. As a result, out-of-range laboratory values were not indicated in the CRF.

Some data in the patient records were written in pencil. CRFs were very neatly written in blue ink. (Black in a medical document would have indicated that the patient had died.) The local culture apparently would not have allowed a CRF with corrections: thus, if there was an error in completion of the CRF, the CRF was destroyed and a new one was completed.

The database listing did not include any adverse events. The CRO indicated that it considered that this information would emerge from review of the progression of the disease. A draft publication which the auditors were asked to review made no mention of adverse events.

CHAPTER 4
Monitoring and Safety Reporting

The conduct of clinical studies is a co-operative undertaking between the sponsor/CRO and the investigator: each is responsible for ensuring that the study is in conformity with the protocol and in accordance with all applicable laws and regulations and, of course, that study subjects are protected at all times. This responsibility involves regular and conscientious review of the progress of the study by the investigator and study site personnel.

One of the most important means of quality control of a clinical study is undertaken by the process of frequent and thorough monitoring. The monitor's aim is to protect the agenda of the sponsor/CRO. Monitors (often referred to as CRAs or clinical research associates or assistants in the pharmaceutical industry) must ensure maintenance of proper standards, compliance with the protocol, accurate and complete data capture and standardisation across sites in a multicentre study. It is a demanding job. Study site personnel should welcome a conscientious monitor who visits on a frequent basis as this can only add to the quality of the study (section 4.1).

Protocol violations and protocol amendments occur during the monitoring period and can have a serious impact on eligibility and evaluability. It is important to appreciate the differences between these terms and understand how to avoid protocol violations and how to manage protocol amendments (section 4.2).

An issue over which site personnel and monitors will be ever watchful is the observation and recording of safety information. In most studies, safety information is under-reported because of the tendency to make judgements which are often based on subjective and biased clinical opinion. It seems difficult to teach clinical researchers to operate as 'scientists': that is, record all observations before making judgements (section 4.3). (This section might also have been included in Chapter 6 as part of data review, but it is important that all personnel realise the importance of capturing data about safety events immediately as they occur.)

4.1   MONITORING

In general, study sites should be visited by a monitor at least every four to six weeks. The frequency of monitoring visits will be defined for each individual study and will depend on details such as the study phase, treatment interval and overall duration, enrolment rate, complexity of the study methodology, occurrence of AEs or other significant events and the nature of the study medication/device. At the beginning of a study, monitoring may be even more intense. In our audit database, monitoring visits by the sponsor/CRO were not adequately frequent (that is, they were greater than two months apart and/or there were less than six visits in one year) at 30% of 378 sites. (This finding probably accounts for the poor quality of data noted elsewhere in this chapter and Chapter 5.)

Each monitoring visit should be preceded by a review by the monitor of the study progress to date and previous monitor reports. The monitor must also consider the impact of any new publications, final study reports, and updates of investigator brochures. If necessary, any new information must be considered for communication to the study site personnel. The monitor will contact the study site to schedule the monitoring visit and determine if there are any particular issues which need to be addressed before the visit, and will usually confirm the proposed visit (date, time and place) by letter, including a copy of an agenda, a list of personnel to be visited, and a list of documents/places to be reviewed. The monitor will plan the monitoring visit to ensure that the investigator and other site personnel will be available for the visit, sufficient time will be available for the needs of the study to be addressed, CRFs and relevant supporting source documents will be available and the storage and dispensing area for the study medication/device will be accessible.

To document appropriate delegation of study site responsibilities and the personal involvement in the study of the nominated investigators, it is necessary that time be allowed to discuss some findings (e.g. protocol violations, CRF entry errors, AEs, problems in recruitment, etc.) with the investigator at every visit. Although it is not necessary for the investigator to be present at all times during the monitoring visits, it is necessary that the investigator be available for some discussion as he/she has ultimate responsibility for the study and clinical care of the study subjects. It is occasionally acceptable for a monitoring visit to occur in the absence of the investigator, but this must be the exceptional situation.

During the monitoring visit at study sites, the monitor will undertake the review noted in Checklist 4.1–1. The most time-consuming task at the study site is the review of source documents to confirm entries in CRFs and compliance with the protocol. This will be further discussed in Chapter 5.

If a CRO and/or a central clinical laboratory is being employed by the sponsor, it is the responsibility of the assigned sponsor's monitor to maintain contact with the CRO and the clinical laboratory on a regular and frequent basis to ensure that the study is being conducted in accordance with the contract. Contacts with the CRO should be at least weekly (and will probably be much more frequent at the beginning of the study) and contacts with the central laboratory should be at least monthly (and again will probably be much more frequent when the study is being set up). The monitor will record observations about the conduct of the CRO and clinical laboratory during the study, and will particularly address the items in Checklist 4.1–2.

A monitoring visit report must be completed by the monitor for each visit to each site of a study, within a specified period (e.g. five working days) of the visit. Significant events (e.g. protocol violations leading to ineligibility or SAEs) must be reported immediately to the sponsor/CRO's designated medical adviser, even if the monitoring report has not yet been completed. Any urgent issues should be immediately communicated by telephone. Telephone contacts may also be completed between visits; however, telephone contacts cannot substitute for visits – the monitor cannot conduct source data verification over the telephone. Further information about the conduct of the study may be in letters of correspondence. Visit reports, telephone contact reports and all other correspondence will also be archived by the sponsor/CRO and investigators will also be required to maintain most of these documents as well. Any information which might be legally sensitive (e.g. information suggesting negligence or fraud on the part of the investigator or the study site), should not be recorded in the monitoring visit reports. Instead, this information should be documented separately and handled confidentially.

At the conclusion of each monitoring visit, the monitor must follow up on any outstanding items (e.g. necessity to send new supplies, updates of the investigator brochure, resolve queries, send new information to the ethics committees/IRBs or regulatory authority, etc.). Before leaving the study site, the monitor should sign and date a list of monitoring visits, maintained at the study site, at each monitoring visit. If other sponsor/CRO personnel visit the study site, they should also sign the visit list, indicating the purpose of their visit. This record, besides providing evidence of sponsor/CRO surveillance during the study, is also an indicator of who had access to confidential information, in case a study subject inquired in the future.

A topic of great interest to managers and monitors is the number of study sites which can be managed by a single monitor. Regular site visits probably take at least a day each, and time to prepare for the visit, to travel to the site and write up a report after a visit must be considered: thus it is unlikely that a monitor can handle more than 10 active study sites given that there are probably numerous internal meetings to attend, that there are only approximately 20 working days in the month and that investigators are not always available on the days planned for the monitoring visit. Of course, the complexity of the study and the recruitment rate influence this number. Today, many companies report that monitors handle a maximum of between five and ten sites. This seems like a reasonable workload given the demands of the job.

. . . A study of an anticoagulant, Italy, 10 patients
The 'CRO' was an academic unit which had no monitors: the investigators reported that they themselves acted as monitors. The first 'monitoring visit' did not occur until seven months after the study had started. Investigators cannot monitor themselves: there must be a degree of independence between those doing the task and those checking on the quality of the task.

. . . A study of hormone replacement therapy, France, 19 patients
Two monitors managed 41 study sites. The investigator had not permitted access to source documents. Because of restrictions on access to source documents, the monitors were not conducting source data verification which probably accounts for the fact that they were able to visit so many sites in such a short time period.

. . . A study of alcohol dependence, Germany, 26 patients
All the CRFs were completed by the monitor. Monitors cannot complete CRFs as monitors work for the sponsor (or the CRO contracted by the sponsor) and thus would be considered to be biased in favour of the sponsor. Further, the investigator is required to include information in CRFs involving 'clinical judgement': it would appear highly unusual if the monitor were to enter such data.

. . . A study of antifungal prophylaxis, UK, 29 patients
The monitor took up to one year to collect CRFs after study treatment had finished. This is a common event. However, data must 'move' promptly as it becomes more and more difficult to resolve discrepancies as the data become older.

When the data have been resolved to the best ability of the monitor (see Chapter 5) and the study has been completed for a particular subject or assessment period, the monitor should retrieve the CRFs for return to the sponsor/CRO, ensuring that the investigator retains a copy. CRFs must be personally collected by the monitor or dispatched by courier directly from the study site, as instructed by the monitor. To minimise risk of loss of CRFs, they should never be sent through the normal mail service, they should never be left in a unlocked car, and they should not be checked in as luggage in the hold on long flights.

The investigator will usually retain the bottom copy of the three-part CRFs; the top two copies will be retrieved by the monitor. Before retrieval, the monitor must ensure that the investigator copy is legible (i.e. that the entry has been copied through from the top copy). Often it is not legible. If it is not legible, the monitor must organise a photocopy to be prepared immediately. CRFs must be retrieved promptly after initial data entry by study site personnel. After retrieval by the sponsor/ CRO, original CRFs should be immediately archived.

Checklist 4.1–1. The Major Objectives of Monitoring Visits

The following tasks should be undertaken by the sponsor/CRO monitor at each study site visit:

- Verify accuracy and completeness of recorded data in CRFs (including diary cards, quality of life forms, registration forms, consent forms, etc.) by comparing with the original source documents (clinic or hospital records). Where discrepancies are found, arrangements must be made for corrections and resolution. Resolve any outstanding queries (ensuring completion of any issued data queries) since the last monitoring visit.

- Verify compliance with entry criteria and procedures, for all study subjects, as specified in the protocol. If subjects are found to be ineligible or unevaluable, these events must be immediately brought to the attention of the investigator as ineligibility and unevaluability may affect the sample size and/or require replacement policies to be considered. There may also be implications for payment to the study site and requirements for reporting to ethics committees/IRBs. Finally, and most seriously, there could be implications for subject safety. The monitor should never instruct the study site to withdraw ineligible subjects unless authorised to do so by the sponsor/CRO's medical adviser or unless there is an immediate threat to the safety of the study subject. (Abrupt withdrawal of some treatments may pose a risk to study subjects.)

- Review all AEs, including clinically significant laboratory abnormalities that have occurred since the previous visit. If a serious or unexpected AE has occurred, which was not correctly reported by the investigator, the monitor must ensure that the correct reporting procedure is followed immediately.

- Evaluate the subject recruitment and withdrawal/dropout rate. If recruitment is less than optimal, suggest ways in which it can be increased. In particular, query the reasons for withdrawals/dropouts, or unscheduled visits, in case these are related to AEs. Ensure that adequate follow-up has occurred for withdrawals/dropouts or that there is documented evidence of attempts to follow up. Ensure that the replacement procedure, if any, is in accordance with the protocol.

- Confirm that all source documents will be retained in a secure location. Source documents must be legible and properly indexed for ease of retrieval. Check the study site file to ensure that all appropriate documents are suitably archived. Provide copies of any missing documents. If extra documents are found at the site which are not in the sponsor/CRO files, these must be copied and retrieved. Check that the investigator files are secure and stored in a separate area which is not accessible to individuals not involved in the study.

- Conduct an inventory and account for study medications/devices and arrange for extra supplies, including other items, such as CRFs, blank forms, etc, if necessary. Resolve discrepancies between inventory and accountability records, and medication/device use, as recorded in the CRFs. If a pharmacy is involved in the study, the pharmacy and pharmacist must be visited. Check that the medication/device is being dispensed in accordance with the protocol. Check that the medication/device is being stored under appropriate environmental conditions and that the expiry dates are still valid. If there is any concern that the medication/device has not been stored properly (e.g. inappropriate exposure to heat, light and humidity) since the last visit or there is no evidence of adequate storage since the last visit, the monitor must report this immediately and document the finding in the monitoring report. Check that the medication/device is securely stored in a separate area that is not accessible to individuals not involved in the study. Check that any supplies shipped to the site since the last visit were received in good condition and are properly stored. If any medications/devices (unused or used containers) must be collected, this should be organised by the monitor at the time of the visit. If applicable, ensure that randomisation procedures are being followed, blind is being maintained, randomisation codebreak envelopes are intact (sealed and stored properly) and a chronological sequence of allocation to treatment is being followed.

• Verify correct clinical sample collection (especially number, type and timing), correct procedures for assays (if applicable), and labelling, storage and transportation of specimens or samples. All clinical laboratory reports should be checked for identification details, validity and continued applicability of reference ranges, accuracy of transcription to CRFs (if any), comments on all out-of-range data and investigator signatures and dates. The dates of sample collection, receipt, analysis and reporting should be checked to ensure that samples are analysed promptly, investigators are informed of results and review them promptly.

• Ensure continued acceptability of facilities, staff and equipment. Ensure that the reference range, documentation of certification and proficiency testing, licensing, and accreditation, for the clinical laboratory are still current. Ensure that there have been no changes in the methods of analysis for specific analytes. Document any changes in clinical site personnel, and if changes have occurred, collect new evidence of suitability of new personnel. Ensure that new staff are fully briefed on the requirements of the protocol and study procedures and arrange any training of new personnel, if necessary. Update signature pages. Document any changes in overall facilities and equipment, and if changes have occurred, collect new evidence of suitability, maintenance, calibration and reason for change of new equipment. Check that adequate security of the facilities continues.

• Advise the investigator and other site personnel of any new developments (e.g. protocol amendments, AEs) which may affect the conduct of the study, and ensure that all financial obligations are being met and check the payment schedule.

Checklist 4.1–2. Management of CROs and Clinical Laboratories During Studies

The CRO and the clinical laboratory must be continually assessed (by the sponsor and the sponsor/CRO, respectively), for the following items:

- Changes, if any, in personnel;
- Changes, if any, in equipment;
- Promptness of response and distribution of visit reports;
- Maintenance of quality control systems;
- Promptness of reporting of significant events (e.g. AEs, protocol amendments) to sponsor, study sites, ethics committees and regulatory authorities. (This would mainly apply to the CRO, although the clinical laboratory would be responsible for prompt reporting of clinically significant laboratory events to the sponsor or CRO.)
- Promptness of data flow to and from the investigator sites;
- Proper management of study medication/device (CRO only);
- Changes if any, in the clinical laboratory protocol (clinical laboratory only);
- Changes, if any, in reference ranges (clinical laboratory only);
- Promptness of sample management (clinical laboratory only), with regard to:
  - Receipt
  - Analysis
  - Issue of laboratory report
  - Promptness of reporting significant out-of-range values to sponsor/CRO;
  - Promptness of reporting significant out-of-range values to investigators;
- Maintenance of accreditation and certification (clinical laboratory only).

4.2 PROTOCOL VIOLATIONS AND PROTOCOL AMENDMENTS

Many researchers confuse the terms 'protocol violations' and 'protocol amendments'. Perhaps the easiest way to explain the difference is to stress that violations are not planned changes (hopefully) to the protocol, whereas protocol amendments are planned changes and are enacted through a formal approval process. (If violations are deliberate or planned, a case of fraud should be considered!)

Most studies will have some protocol violations despite

the most meticulous efforts of site personnel and careful monitoring. These events happen simply because people make mistakes and also because it is difficult to write a protocol which foresees every possible event. However, the most serious effect of protocol violations is on eligibility and evaluability and thus violations must be avoided as much as possible. A study is designed to include a sample size which gives meaningful statistical results but which exposes the least number of study subjects possible to the risk of inclusion in a clinical study. (A clinical study must always be considered a risk: the study is being conducted to answer a question for which we do not know the answer (else why undertake the study) and it is usually conducted in the development stages of a product when relatively few individuals have been exposed to treatment.)

... A study of an anticoagulant, UK, 12 patients
One of the main end-points of the study was the number of blood transfusions required for patients undergoing surgery. The investigator entered a Jehovah's witness. The writers of the protocol obviously did not foresee this possibility and thus did not include an appropriate exclusion criterion. It would be highly unlikely that any protocols would include such specific criteria.

Any planned change to an approved protocol must be implemented by a formal protocol amendment. An amendment is required for all changes to the protocol: there is no distinction between minor and major changes, revisions, deviations, etc. although many sponsors/CROs try to make these kinds of distinctions in the hope that it will reduce the volume of paper. The ICH GCP guideline on GCP was helpful in clarifying this point by emphasizing that all protocol changes require review and approval by ethics committees/IRBs. Nevertheless, there is still much 'evasion' on this point. For example, adding new sites to a study, changing investigators and adding new investigators to a site can have a serious impact on studies with regard to homogeneity of the patient population and the variation in medical practice between different investigators. However, few sponsors/CROs prepare amendments for these types of changes in study design.
... A study of breast cancer, Mexico, several sites

The study was being conducted in Europe and North America. As recruitment was slow, the sponsor decided to involve an affiliate office in Mexico. The drug was a cytotoxic agent and expected side effects were alopecia and nausea/vomiting. After the data were compiled, it was noted that the incidence of alopecia was much lower than expected. The sponsor's marketing department was pleased with this finding as the product was to be promoted as more 'gentle'. When the situation was investigated further, it was found that when the study subjects in Mexico presented themselves at the clinics, their heads were immediately shaved: thus, there was no alopecia to report!

... A study of lower respiratory tract infection, Africa, several sites
A study with an oral cephalosporin was being conducted in Europe and North America. As recruitment was slow, the sponsor decided to involve an affiliate office in Africa. The expected side effects revolved around gastrointestinal disturbance. After the data were compiled, it was noted that the incidence of 'diarrhoea' was much lower than expected. When the situation was investigated further, it was found that the study subjects and investigators considered that these events were not AEs: rather, this was a good way of 'cleansing the body'.

Proposed protocol amendments must be circulated to all original signatories of the protocol for review and approval, and protocol amendment approval must be documented. In multicentre studies it is necessary for all sites to consider and implement protocol amendments. Amendments specific to one site (or less than the total number of sites) must be avoided as they may result in confounding results with regard to the major hypothesis as a result of significant inter-site variability which will only be discovered at the end of the study during data analysis. In our audit database, investigators did not sign protocol amendments at 29% of 378 sites.

Protocol amendments can have an impact on other aspects of the study. In particular, it may be necessary to review the CRF, the information sheet and consent form, and the investigator brochure. Protocol amendments may also result in the necessity to reinform study subjects and obtain consent again, and may necessitate consideration by insurance companies, especially if the planned changes include expansion of the study population size or extension of the duration of the clinical study.

After approval by the sponsor/CRO and the investigator, the protocol amendment must be submitted externally to the ethics committees/IRBs (and regulatory authorities, if applicable) for review and approval, before implementation. The final approved protocol amendment must be circulated to all recipients of the final approved protocol. The sponsor/CRO should maintain a list of protocol amendment recipients to assist in accountability of these documents and ensure all holders of the protocol also receive the protocol amendment. At monitoring visits, the monitor should check that protocol amendments are in the investigator's file and are retained with the protocol. Many companies seem to have great difficulties in controlling distribution of protocol amendments. Amendments were not distributed to all recipients of the final protocol at 55% of 226 sites in our audit database.

. . . A study of hormone replacement therapy, The Netherlands, 21 study subjects
Significant changes to the protocol were not adequately managed in a standardised and formalised manner. The following findings indicated a confused situation: the first? 'amendment' was not numbered and referred to two different studies; the investigator did not have a copy of this first? amendment although a signature page was in his files; another 'amendment' (labelled 'change to addendum') was also not numbered and an external signature page was not available; a significant change in study design (cancellation of an extension study because of production and stability problems with the drug) was not formalised in an amendment; and all amendments were not apparently distributed to all recipients of the protocol.

. . . A study of breast cancer, Canada, six patients
Four amendments to the protocol were accompanied by a letter stating that they should not be regarded as amendments!

. . . A study of cardiovascular surgery, France, 28 patients
Protocol amendments were not approved by ethics committees because the consultative committees (basically ethics committees in France) had

been dissolved owing to new regulations in France.

... A study of hypertension, Germany, 32 patients
The study started out with 24 sites, as specified in the protocol. Eventually 34 sites were involved and there was no protocol amendment. One site decided to do kinetic studies unilaterally: no amendment was prepared.

Checklist 4.2–1. Contents of Protocol Amendments

Each protocol amendment should indicate:
- Protocol amendment number;
- Protocol title, number and date;
- Date of approval of amendment;
- Issue date (e.g. the date on which the protocol amendment takes effect after approval);
- Protocol amendment text: this must be a clear statement of the words, lines, paragraphs or pages of the protocol that are being changed. Both the original text that is being changed and the new text must be stated.
- Reason for protocol amendment;
- Signatures: the required signatories will be indicated on this page. Each dated signature will include the name (in capital letters), title and date of the signature. The date must be entered by the signatory.

4.3   REPORTING AND RECORDING SAFETY EVENTS

All adverse events (AEs), serious, unexpected or minor, occurring during clinical studies must be recorded in CRFs, their significance must be assessed and other information must be provided for reporting AEs externally (e.g. to regulatory authorities and ethics committees/IRBs). This applies to any study treatment (including comparator agents, placebo and non-medical therapy) and any stage of the study (e.g. run-in, washout, active treatment, follow-up) whether or not the medication/device is marketed by the sponsor/CRO. The monitor and all clinical research personnel must ensure that all safety information is documented.

The sponsor/CRO will be responsible for ensuring that the investigator and her/his staff are fully educated with regard to reporting of all AEs. Site personnel must be instructed to observe and record information prior to making judgements about the information and they must be taught to search for clues about safety events from many sources such as information in source documents at the study sites; information in data collection forms (e.g. CRFs, diary cards, quality of life forms, psychiatric rating scales, etc.); occurrence of missed and/or unscheduled visits, dropouts and withdrawals; use of any concomitant medications/devices; and abnormal laboratory data. AEs may also result simply as a result of study procedures and study participation. Information about definitions of AEs and requirements for reporting AEs (Checklists 4.3–1 and 4.3–2) must be clearly stated in the protocol and explained to the investigator staff at the initiation meetings. All investigators and investigator staff will also be educated in the correct procedure and immediate requirement for reporting of serious adverse events (SAEs) and/or unexpected AEs to the sponsor/CRO.

Our audit database shows that there is significant under-reporting of safety information in many clinical studies. Safety events were not reported (or inadequately reported) in 41% of 378 study sites. Non-compliance with safety reporting requirements is dangerous for present and future patients. Lack of rigour in reporting safety data is a universal problem and there is definitely a bias against reporting safety data, probably due to factors such as the following: viewing safety data as 'negative' data and therefore not to be reported, the extensive paperwork requirements, poor training of sponsor/CRO and site personnel and overly subjective assessments of safety data (e.g. prejudgement of the significance of certain types of events) by both investigators and sponsor/CRO personnel.

As soon as CRFs are retrieved from the study site by the sponsor/CRO, a designated sponsor/CRO person must review the CRFs for safety issues. All CRFs containing AEs should be further reviewed to ensure that SAEs are correctly and promptly reported to ethics committees/IRBs and regulatory authorities. The monitor will seek advice from the sponsor/

CRO's medical adviser to ensure that all necessary information is collected promptly to satisfy external reporting requirements.

Although rules for SAE reporting may vary slightly internationally, in general, all SAEs and/or unexpected AEs (including clinical and laboratory events) must be reported immediately (e.g. within 24–48 hours) to the sponsor/CRO's medical adviser as soon as notification is received by the monitor or otherwise noted by any staff member during the review of the CRFs. SAEs must be assessed by a medically qualified person employed or contracted by the sponsor/CRO. The emergency contact numbers of the sponsor/CRO medical adviser should be noted in the protocol and should be easily available on a 24-hour basis.

The reporting of SAEs must be documented by the investigator on a special SAE report form, which is usually prepared by the sponsor/CRO so that it addresses all regulatory requirements. A copy of the CRF, if completed, should be attached to the SAE form. Information for the proper description and evaluation of a SAE may not be available within the required time frame after first learning of the event. Follow-up must continue until the event is resolved or the condition is unlikely to change or is lost to follow-up: all events must have closure.

Some other important points to remember with regard to SAE reporting include: if a SAE is considered to be drug-related by the investigator, but is not considered to be drug-related by the sponsor/CRO (or vice versa), the event must be treated as drug-related for the purposes of reporting to regulatory authorities; in the case of blind studies, the medical adviser (and the investigator) may, if necessary, break the randomisation code to identify the test substance (a procedure which must be fully documented, see Chapter 6); and any information presented in SAE reports must be treated with confidentiality. Study subject names must not be divulged. (Many investigators submit reports with full patient names which are then retained in the sponsor/CRO archives.) These procedures also apply to any other SAE noted by a member of the clinical research department during the conduct of duties. The events may arise from the following sources: spontaneous reports from research subjects, study site personnel or members of the public; post-marketing surveillance; other companies; and published literature.

All investigators and other study site personnel, ethics committees/IRBs and possibly study subjects, must be informed of all new significant safety information by the sponsor/CRO, including all events occurring with any treatment (e.g. washout, investigational product, comparator, placebo, etc.) in the study, even if these occurred in another study with the same treatment, or in another country. Significant safety information includes all SAEs and any other events (e.g. significant trends in laboratory data or new preclinical data) which might have an impact on the risk assessment of the study. Information about SAEs may only be reported externally after formal authorisation by the sponsor/CRO medical adviser. Reporting to other groups (e.g. co-operative oncology groups, steering committees, special safety panels) must also be considered. As a minimum standard, all SAEs which are reported to regulatory authorities must also be reported to the groups noted above. The monitor must ensure that the investigator has fulfilled the obligation to report to local ethics committees/IRBs.

Safety events may necessitate an update to the investigator brochure, the protocol and CRF, and the information sheet and consent form. The sponsor/CRO medical adviser is also responsible for reporting safety events occurring during preclinical studies and following through with the consequences (e.g. changes in development plan, requirement to inform study site personnel, necessity to discontinue clinical studies, etc.). If the safety events require modification or discontinuation of the study, all investigators must be informed quickly (e.g. within one working day) and if it is necessary to recall clinical study supplies, the procedures described in Chapter 6 should be followed. Additionally, regulatory authorities and ethics committees/IRBs must be informed.

Safety summaries, including listings of all SAEs, will be prepared by the sponsor/CRO clinical research department. The summary must include a description of any changes in the estimate of risk to the study subjects receiving the study medication/device. Further, the sponsor/CRO is responsible for reviewing final clinical reports to ensure that all safety data are fully and accurately reported. Reporting safety events related to a marketed comparator must also be considered: the sponsor/

CRO has the responsibility to report to the company authorised to market the comparator, but not necessarily to the local regulatory authorities (depending on local regulations).

... A study of hypertension, Germany, 32 patients
All *'severe'* AEs were considered to be *'serious'*. Many sponsor/CRO and site personnel do not recognise the distinction between 'severe' and 'serious'.

... A study of the pharmacokinetics of drug X in surgical patients, France, 97 patients
An AE (intense nausea and vomiting) was reported in only one subject which seemed unlikely to the auditors. The investigators said that some other patients reported mild nausea and vomiting: however, in his opinion, patients in France did not usually have these symptoms and therefore he did not think these were important to report! This is a good example of researchers making judgements before recording observations. Several similar examples follow – this is an all too common event.

... A study of the pharmacokinetics of drug X, Finland, 65 paediatric patients
The investigator was instructed (in the protocol) only to report AEs which she considered to be important. No AEs were reported in CRFs: however, in the small audit sample, the auditors found evidence of several AEs reported in clinical notes. The protocol provided the wrong instructions – a common occurrence.

... A study of drug X administered by injection, Spain, 32 patients
In correspondence with the sponsor, the investigator reported that many patients suffered pain, redness and swelling at the injection site which was more than expected. This AE was not recorded in any CRFs and thus was not reflected in the database listing or reported in the final clinical study report.

... A study of an anxiolytic, UK, eight patients
A senior representative of the pharmaceutical company was of the opinion that AEs occurring during a run-in period should not be reported as AEs in the CRFs. There was evidence of several AEs occurring during this period which were not recorded on the database.

Similar AEs occurring during the treatment phase were recorded as new events although they were actually continuations of previously existing events. This situation underlines the importance of obtaining a detailed baseline assessment.

... A study of an anticoagulant, Denmark, 13 patients
Although a 35 day follow-up period was required by the protocol, AEs were required to be followed only up for the first seven days of the study in the CRF.

... A study of an anticoagulant, Australia, 36 patients
Three SAEs (including two deaths) were noted in the clinical records by the auditors. The SAEs were not reported because the sponsor did not consider them to be related to the study drug.

... A study of hormone replacement therapy, Canada, 13 study subjects
The company used quality of life forms which were 'symptom-driven', that is the forms posed questions to study subjects about the intensity of 'expected' symptoms. Many patients reported severe events of hot flushes, sweating attacks, aching joints/muscles, stiffness of limbs, vaginal dryness, pain on intercourse, bloated feeling, back pains, abdominal cramps, backache, nausea, sore breasts, palpitations, head-aches, neck pains, etc. Many of the symptoms also worsened during the study. None of these events were listed as AEs in the database. Data listings will appear unconvincing if listings of AEs are not consistent with listings of data derived from quality of life forms, diary cards, rating scales, use of concomitant medications, etc.

... A study of diabetes, Canada, 22 patients
SAE reports were signed by the monitor and the study site co-ordinator. The study co-ordinator, who was a nurse, was indicated as the treating physician on the SAE report. Data collection forms of any type should never be completed by monitors or other sponsor/ CRO personnel. All SAE reports need the attention of the designated physician-investigator.

... A study of stroke, Portugal, 500 patients
No SAEs were reported over a four-year period. The auditors found this difficult to believe in a population which had previously suffered

strokes. In fact, source data verification had not been permitted during the study and thus the monitor had not been able to verify safety reporting.

... A study of intensive care patients, UK, three sites
At one site (18 patients recruited), three patients died during the study. At another site (15 patients recruited), four patients died during the study. At the third site (11 patients recruited), seven patients died during the study. None of the deaths were reported as SAEs and none of the events appeared in the database.

Checklist 4.3-1. Adverse Event Terminology

The following definitions of adverse event terminology should be understood by all clinical research participants:
- Adverse Event: An adverse event (AE) is any untoward medical occurrence in a patient or clinical investigation subject administered a pharmaceutical product and which does not necessarily have a causal relational with this treatment (ICH, 1994).
- Adverse drug reaction: all noxious and unintended responses to a medical product related to any dose should be considered an adverse drug reaction (ADR) (ICH, 1994). (The term 'adverse drug reaction' (ADR) is normal terminology used in the literature. However, the term 'adverse reaction' might be better used in SOPs to reflect consideration of both medications and devices.)
- Unexpected adverse drug reaction: an adverse reaction, the nature or severity of which is not consistent with applicable product labelling (e.g. the investigator brochure for an approved experimental drug; the data sheet (or product monograph) for a marketed product) (ICH, 1994);
- Serious adverse event: a serious adverse event or reaction is an untoward medical occurrence that at any dose (ICH, 1994 and FDA, Federal Register, 1994):
  - Results in death;
  - Is life-threatening;
  - Requires inpatient hospitalization or prolongation of existing hospitalisation;
  - Results in persistent or significant disability/incapacity;

- Leads to any congenital anomaly;
- Necessitates medical or surgical intervention to preclude perma-nent impairment of a body function or permanent damage to body structure.
- Minor adverse event: all AEs which are not considered to be serious or unexpected may be described as 'minor' for the purposes of reporting. (This is not a regulatory definition: only a suggested definition.)

The relationship of an AE to the study medication/device should be graded as follows (this is a suggested scheme: the regulatory documents do not specify how 'relationship' should be graded):

- None: the AE is definitely not associated with the study medication/device administered.
- Remote: the temporal association is such that the study medication/device is not likely to have had an association with the observed AE.
- Possible: this causal relationship is assigned when the AE: (a) follows a reasonable temporal sequence from medication/device administration, but (b) could have been produced by the study subject's clinical state or other modes of therapy administered to the study subject.
- Probable: this causal relationship is assigned when the AE (a) follows a reasonable temporal sequence from medication/device administration, (b) abates upon discontinuation of the treatment (c) cannot be reasonably explained by known characteristics of the study subject's clinical state.
- Highly probable: this causal relationship is assigned when the AE (a) follows a reasonable temporal sequence from medication/device administration, (b) abates upon discontinuation of the treatment and (c) is confirmed by reappearance of the AE on repeat exposure (rechallenge).

The severity (or intensity) of AEs should be assessed according to the following definitions (this is a suggested scheme: the regulatory documents do not specify how 'severity' should be graded):

- Mild: the AE is transient, requires no treatment, and does not inter-fere with the study subject's daily activities.
- Moderate: the AE introduces a low level of inconvenience or concern to the study subject and may interfere with daily activities, but is usually ameliorated by simple therapeutic measures.

- Severe: the AE interrupts the study subject's usual daily activity and requires systematic therapy or other treatment.

Checklist 4.3–2. Items of Information to Include on AE Pages in CRFs

Information which should be included on the AE page in CRFs includes:
- Study site identification;
- Study subject number/code;
- Visit date;
- Visit number;
- Description of AE;
- Type/symptoms;
- Date and time of first occurrence;
- Continuous or intermittent;
- Stop date and time;
- Intensity (e.g. mild, moderate, severe);
- Relationship to study medication/device (e.g. none, remote, possible, probable, highly probable);
- Action taken (e.g. none, concomitant treatment, other);
- Outcome (e.g. recovered, continuing, fatal, unknown);
- Requirement to indicate whether or not the AE was serious;
- Requirement to indicate whether or not the AE was unexpected;
- Instructions for further reporting, if serious or unexpected.

CASE STUDY FOUR

A Single-Centre Double-Blind Study to Investigate the Effect of Drug X in Approximately 50 Patients Undergoing Bypass Surgery (Europe).

The lack of reporting of safety data was the most serious issue in this study, which had been completed about two years prior to the audit. The investigator stated to the auditors that since the study involved an elderly population which would be expected to encounter serious health problems, he did not think the

> *safety events were worth reporting to the sponsor (and clearly the sponsor did not try to verify the safety reports). However, there were many other problems with this study as well. What would you do to rectify this situation? The auditors only met with a junior physician during the audit – the investigator who had signed the protocol was not available.*

Summary of Major Deficiencies

Standard Operating Procedures: The SOPs were not comprehensive: many important topics were not addressed (e.g. training and qualification of sponsor personnel, investigator agreements, study site initiation, source data verification procedures, randomisation procedures, study medication/device requisition, packaging and labelling, shipment, control at the study site, disposition/destruction, auditing and inspection).

Ethics Committee Review: The study started out as a single centre and a second centre was later added (there was no protocol amendment) although the auditors could not determine which patients were entered at which centre. The approval letter from the ethics committee predated the final protocol date and referred to an 'outline protocol' which consisted of three pages. There was no indication that the ethics committee had reviewed many important required items prior to granting approval to conduct the study (e.g. adequacy of confidentiality protection, payments to the investigator, insurance for the protection of the study subject, CRF, investigator brochure, suitability of investigator and facilities, number of study subjects at each site and justification for the sample size). There was no record of any ongoing review by the ethics committee. In particular, the committee had not been informed of the occurrence of at least three SAEs which were noted by the auditors during a review of a sample of CRFs. The details of the membership of the ethics committees were inadequate and the auditors were unable to assess the lists to determine any conflicts of interest. The membership list for ethics committee A was obtained three years after the start of the study (and was dated three years after the start of the study).

Informed Consent Procedures: The consent form and information sheet were inadequate in content. In particular, the following important items were missing: direct access to source documents to be required, description of the study medication, procedures to be followed, correct explanation of duration of participation, known risks of the medication, inadequate description of compensation, emergency contact number and family doctor to be informed of participation. There was no evidence that revision of the consent form was considered after the occurrence of the SAEs.

There were several irregularities in the consent procedure. The consent procedure was not undertaken by authorised investigators. A non-physician was obtaining consent for some subjects. The subjects were not dating the consent forms themselves. All 'investigators' signed in the place allocated for the witness, but there was no witness to the consent procedure in this study. Four investigator signatures were unidentifiable. Consent from some subjects was obtained after the start of treatment. In two cases, the date for the patient's signature had been overwritten by an unidentifiable individual: the original dates postdated study entry while the corrected dates predated the study entry.

Protocol: There were many deficiencies in the protocol approval process: there was no evidence of any internal (sponsor) approval of the protocol; the protocol was signed only by the 'principal' investigator, although research fellows were actually conducting the study; the first study subject received treatment at least four months prior to documented approval (by the sponsor, investigator, or the ethics committees) of the final protocol; the protocol signature page was apparently added to the protocol several months after the issue of the protocol; and the investigator did not have a copy of the protocol signature page.

The protocol was missing many important items (e.g. statistician review, preclinical summary and background to the study, study design, number of study sites, proposed duration of study, total number of study subjects to be recruited and to be considered evaluable, procedures to ensure and assess compliance with study medication and to modify the study and manage protocol amendments, justification for the dose, labelling, packaging, storage, instructions for safe handling and disposal of study medications, requirements for maintaining accountability records, identification of clinical laboratory and management of samples, procedures for reporting SAEs, management of clinically significant laboratory values, randomisation procedures, monitoring and methods of data verification, instructions for completion and correction of CRFs, type and scope of planned statistical analysis, justification for the sample size and criteria for evaluability of safety and effectiveness).

The protocol was also misleading in some respects. For example, the protocol implied that the study was a Phase IV study since it was 'being given at the dosage and for the indications described in the product licence'. However, the protocol also stated that 'no studies have been undertaken to investigate the potential protective effect of Drug X in patients undergoing bypass surgery'. On page x, the protocol indicated that there would be an assessment at a minimum of six months post-operatively: on page y, the protocol indicated that there would be 26 weeks of oral treatment post-operatively. In the CRF, 48 weeks of treatment were indicated: the information sheet indicated that treatment would be up to one year. Although a laboratory safety screen was not required for this study, most subjects had undergone these assessments before, during and after the study. There were no instructions in the protocol for assessing these items, and to report AEs if changes in laboratory values were considered to be clinically significantly abnormal.

CRF Design: The CRF design did not allow for the collection of all required information (e.g. study centre identification, visit date, duration of medical condition, medical history, previous and concomitant treatments, details of study medication administration, clinical laboratory data, and several important details for safety data). The design (single-page format) did not allow for secure retrieval and transmission of data. The CRF requirements (e.g. demographics, selection criteria, physical examination) did not always match the protocol. The CRF sign off (by the investigator) requirement was inadequate: it was only necessary to sign-off at the end of the entire treatment period.

Setting Up the Study: An investigator brochure was not present at the beginning of the study and it was not updated during the study. (The brochure was provided to the investigators three years after the start of the study.) The investigator brochure did not contain information about the disposal of the study medication or the management of accidental exposure. No information was provided about the placebo comparator.

There was no documentation of the qualifications of the study monitor or any other sponsor personnel involved in the study. There was no indication that the monitor had obtained documentation of the training and qualifications of the investigators at the start of the study. CVs obtained after the start of the study did not indicate previous experience in clinical research or GCP. There was no documentation (for site personnel) of other current clinical research commitments and availability of adequate time for the study. There was no evidence that the study site was formally assessed prior to placement of the study and there was no record of an initiation visit. A sponsor/investigator contract was signed five months after the first subject entered the study and did not adequately describe investigator responsibilities.

Monitoring: Up to three months after the start of the study, there was no formal standardised record of monitoring visits and some previous letters describing monitoring activities were not signed or dated. The overall frequency of monitoring was inadequate. The monitor reports were missing some important items of assessment and given the number of errors noted by the auditors in a small sample of CRFs (see below), it did not appear that source data verification was conducted.

Control of Clinical Study Medication: The request for shipment preceded the date on which the investigator signed the final protocol. There was no record of the actual shipment of study medication to the study site or receipt of study medication in the study files.

The study medication labels were missing important information (e.g. the statement that medication was for clinical purposes only). The instructions on the labels were to store the medication below 20 °C; however, the investigator brochure stated that the medication should be stored below 25 °C. The temperature in the pharmacy was not apparently controlled or monitored, according to the pharmacist. There was a temperature-reporting device, which was observed as 22 °C by the auditors.

The dispensing records in the pharmacy were missing some important information. In particular, returns of used containers were not documented: the pharmacy reported that this was the responsibility of the investigator, but he did not have any records of return and disposal. There was no evidence of an ongoing inventory (a running balance) of the study medication. The record of returns retained by the sponsor did not reconcile with the dispensing records and CRF entries.

The study blind was compromised. The monitor apparently generated the randomisation code and thus was fully aware of treatment allocation. A list of the randomisation assignments was openly available to the monitor in the study file. The correct sequence of treatment allocation was not followed (i.e. patients were not randomised to treatment in order).

Filing/Archiving: All original documents were still in working files at the sponsor site (several years after the start of the study). No documents were retained in secure archives. The investigator records were not secure: they were located in three different offices with no apparent restrictions on access. Some important documents were missing from both the investigator and sponsor archives.

Source Data: CRFs were not available for all subjects at the sponsor and investigator sites. Although there were approximately 50 subjects in the study, the sponsor could only locate 41 CRFs for the auditors and the investigator could only locate 36. He checked at his home as well as the offices on the day of the audit. One CRF was not available at either location, although there was evidence that study medication had been used for this subject. Additionally, source documents (medical charts) for two of the six subjects in the audit sample were not available. The hospital was unable to locate the records, although notification of the impending audit had been issued several weeks earlier: the hospital personnel were still trying to locate the records on the day of the audit.

There was no evidence that primary care physicians had been informed of study participation. (The investigator reported that he had notified family doctors but had not retained any evidence of this.)

There were several discrepancies, with regard to fulfilment of selection criteria, when comparing the CRFs and source documents. Some examples of discrepancies in the audit sample were:

Subject x: The medical records indicated that the subject had glaucoma, but CRF page x did not indicate any abnormalities of the eyes.

Subject x: On CRF page x, there was no indication of whether or not the subject had a previous myocardial infarction, although this was in the source documents. The investigator reported no history of angina in the CRF, but the source documents indicated that there was a history of angina. The patient also apparently suffered from asthma and a cataract in the left eye. None of these events were reported in the CRF. The investigator recorded a 'chronically sore toe' but did not indicate abnormality of the extremities on CRF page x.

Subject x: No abnormalities were ticked on CRF page x, but other comments indicated 'ischaemia of the left foot'.

Subject x: No abnormalities were ticked on CRF page x, but other comments indicated 'gangrenous toe'.

The source documents did not clearly indicate all visit dates and exposure to the study medication. The date (but not the time) of the start of infusion could be determined in some cases, but details of continuation of the infusion was not always evident. Issue and use of oral medication was not always clearly recorded. Some examples of discrepancies in the audit sample were:

Subject x: Apparently visits 1 and 2 both occurred on the same day. Was it possible to determine all eligibility criteria in this time interval?

Subject x: The day of surgery was recorded as x in the source summary notes, but apparently the surgery occurred three days earlier according to the surgical procedure notes.

Subject x: On CRF page x (no subject number was on this page, but it was attached to other pages with this subject number), the investigator indicated that the subject had not completed the full study period. He then completed the CRF page as though the subject had finished the full study.

There were several discrepancies, with regard to concomitant medication use. Several medications reported in the source documents during the study period were not recorded in the CRF. Some examples of discrepancies in the audit sample were:

Subject x: The subject received aspirin during and post-operatively: this medication was prohibited by the protocol. The medical records also clearly indicated in several places that this individual was sensitive to aspirin.

Subject x: On CRF page x, aspirin was noted as a concomitant medication, but the indication was not recorded.

There were numerous inconsistencies in reporting AEs. Many AEs noted in source documents were not recorded in CRFs. Some examples of discrepancies in the audit sample were:

Subject x: This subject died during the study, but a SAE report was not completed.

Subject x: There were comments in the CRF about a 'rash', but this was not reported as an AE.

Subject x: There were comments in the CRF about 'nausea', but the AE form was not completed.

Subject x: At visit x, the investigator reported YES for AEs, but a form had not been completed. There were no details of AEs.

Subject x: On CRF page x, the investigator commented 'pt unwell': no AE form was completed. In the source medical records, 'itchy lesions', 'widespread erythema', 'rash perseveres' were recorded during the study period: AE forms were not completed.

Subject x: 'Flushing/dizziness' was recorded at Visits x and x, but an AE form was not completed.

Subject x: This patient died during the study period, but a SAE form was not completed. Post-operatively, 'lots of vomiting' was recorded in the medical notes with an indication that it might be due to 'drug X' (study medication). On Post-operative day x, 'nausea' was reported in the medical notes. Several other events ('aspiration pneumonia', 'collapse', 'heart failure', 'amputation') were recorded in the source documents, but none of these were reported as AEs in the CRF. At visit x in the CRF, the investigator had reported no AEs. Previous to this date, the source documents indicated that the 'emergency arrest team' had been called out and CPR 'had been carried out for 2–3 minutes'. Comments in the CRF (page x) indicated that the subject had undergone a second amputation. This could not be verified in the source documents. A SAE form had not been completed.

Subject x: The randomisation code envelope was required to be opened because of significant post-operative bleeding – not reported as an AE in the CRF.

Subject x: At Visit x, the investigator reported 'NO' for AEs, yet commented that there was a 'minor vein irritation'. (An AE form was not completed.)

Subject x: At Visit x, the investigator commented in the CRF 'bleeding poorly at night – probably unrelated to medication'. The event was not reported as an AE.

Subject x: At Visit x, the investigator ticked YES in the CRF for AEs. No symptoms were specified. An AE form was not completed.

Subject x: Several comments were noted in the CRF (including a 'below knee amputation'). An AE form was not completed.

Three deaths were noted in records at the sponsor site, but these were not recorded as SAEs. In addition to the three deaths, new deaths and hospitalisations were noted during the study period in the audit sample. No events were formally reported as SAEs.

The CRF photocopies provided to the auditors were not always legible. Extra CRF data entries (not required by the CRF layout) were numerous. These entries were not clearly flagged and their significance was not assessed. CRFs were not signed and dated by authorised investigators. For seven subjects, the CRFs were signed by a non-physician. In some cases the signatures were entered three to five months after study completion.

The data correction procedure at the study site was inadequate. All data corrections were not clearly indicated, dated and initialled, and they were not authorised by the investigator. Original data entries were sometimes obscured. Data query forms had not been issued, even though data had been entered several years previously. Data review was not prompt. The monitor did not retrieve CRFs within a reasonable interval of their completion by the investigator and the sponsor did not review CRFs within a reasonable interval of their retrieval by the monitor. The sponsor did not enter CRF data on the predefined computerised database within a reasonable interval of their retrieval by the monitor. Apparently no data had yet been computerised at the time of the audit.

CHAPTER 5
Collecting Data with Integrity

Collecting data that are accurate, honest, reliable and credible is one of the most important and one of the most difficult objectives of conducting clinical research.

At the study site, the main means of verifying data is by meticulous monitoring. The monitor must determine, by review of source documents, that the data submitted to the sponsor/CRO in the CRFs and other data collection forms are reliable. Data in CRFs are not credible to the regulators unless they can be supported by the 'real' documents (i.e.the source documents maintained at the study site for the clinical care of the study subject). To undertake the process of source data verification, the monitors must have direct access to source documents at the study site. Most sponsors and CROs have great difficulties determining how far they must go in the verification process and thus it is necessary to have a sensible plan which encourages site personnel to maintain good records (sections 5.1– 5.3).

After data are retrieved from the study site, there are further means of assessing those data. First, there is the initial review at the sponsor/CRO premises after retrieval from the study sites: this process is sometimes referred to as secondary monitoring. Thereafter, review by the data management department is another extremely important means of quality control. It is a lengthy and complex process and there are few guidelines and regulations for reference. (We will only address a few points in this chapter which directly involve the monitor and the study site personnel, as this topic is otherwise worthy of a much more detailed approach.) These processes will inevitably result in queries about the data. To ensure that the integrity of clinical research data is maintained and that there is total agreement between the data recorded on CRFs, the data entered on the computer, the data recorded in data listings and cross tabulations, the data entered into statistical and clinical study reports, and finally the data in the sponsor/CRO and investigator archives, it is essential that the data must only be changed by following a formal procedure. Finally, there will be statistical input into management of the data. Although most clinical research personnel will not have the necessary expertise to make statistical evaluations, they should understand basic statistical requirements (sections 5.4–5.6).

5.1   THE DIFFERENCE BETWEEN SOURCE DOCUMENTS AND CRFS

Source documents (and the data contained therein) comprise the following types of documents: patient files (medical notes where summaries of physical examination findings, details of medical history, concurrent medications/devices and diseases are noted), recordings from automated instruments, traces (ECG, EEG), X-ray films, laboratory notes and computer databases (e.g. psychological tests requiring direct entry by patient on to computers or direct entry of patient information on to computers by physicians).

CRFs are documents designed by the researchers to collect research data. It is important that CRFs only collect data necessary for the research question – collecting too few or too many data might be unethical or unscientific – and thus the CRF is a biased document in the sense that only data which are relevant to the proposed hypothesis will be collected.

The primary purpose of source documents is for the care of the study subject from a clinical perspective: the primary purpose of CRFs is to collect research data. CRFs (and other data collection forms) generally cannot substitute as source documents. Data entered in CRFs should generally be supported by source data in source documents, except as specifically defined at the beginning of the study. Nevertheless, some data entered in CRFs may be source data (e.g. voluminous blood pressure readings, numerous psychiatric rating scales, etc.) and would not be found elsewhere. This may be acceptable if these data would not normally be entered in medical records, and if knowledge of such data is not required by the investigator or other clinicians who concurrently or subsequently treat the study subject. (The protocol should specify which data will be source data in the CRF.)

Before each study begins, a meeting of sponsor/CRO personnel must be held to assess each CRF entry field and determine whether or not the CRF entry is expected to be directly supported by entries in source documents. The monitor, in particular, should be provided with written instructions regarding the source of data. Subsequently the investigator and site personnel should be informed as to the minimum expectations for source data verification, and should be given clear instructions as to what information will be necessary in the source documents. The results of this discussion should be documented in the pre-study assessment visit report and in the study site initiation report.

If source data are entered directly on to a computer, there must be a safeguard to ensure validation, including a signed and dated printout to use as backup records. In fact, at each visit, the monitor should obtain a printout, which is signed and dated by the investigator, and which serves as the source document and is maintained at the study site. This process is necessary because most clinical settings do not have systems which are sophisticated enough to provide a secure and accurate data audit trail, that is, a trail of when and how data are changed, if at all, and have not been reliably validated (i.e. have SOPs and procedures to ensure the survival of the electronic data).

... A study of hypertension, UK, 21 patients
The investigator reported that source documents were not available as they were normally sent home with the patients who were instructed to return them to the clinic at each visit. The investigator explained that

his clinic was very progressive and did not think they needed to retain patient notes!

... A study of an anxiolytic, France, 23 patients
There were no source documents at the study site. The investigator explained that he did not maintain clinical notes – he relied on his memory.

... A study of prostate cancer, UK, 56 patients (two sites)
No source documents were available for 19 subjects and no explanation was provided.

... A study of cardiovascular surgery, UK, six patients
The investigator, who worked alone, did not maintain patient notes. He felt they were unnecessary and that the CRFs were an adequate substitute for source documents. This finding, and the above examples, obviously indicate that source document verification was not undertaken by the study monitor, and therefore the sponsor/ CRO submitted unverified data to the regulatory authorities. Except for the USA, regulators in other countries generally accept these data and ask no further questions – the FDA inspectors would undoubtedly fail these studies if they were to inspect them. Many clinical researchers suggest that the source data verification process indicates that we do not 'trust' researchers and that it should not be undertaken. Unfortunately, experience has taught us that the biases in clinical research and the lack of adequate training in the rigours of maintaining reliable data do indeed mean that poor data are inevitable without the process of source document verification. It is not a matter of lack of trust – it is an indication that much more training in record-keeping is required.

5.2   ACCESS TO SOURCE DOCUMENTS

Direct access to source documents is required for all studies – direct access means monitors, auditors, other authorised representatives of the sponsor/CRO and inspectors are permitted to view all relevant source documents needed to verify the CRF data entries. Other restricted methods of access to source documents (e.g. 'across-the-table', 'back-to-back', 'interview method') are not acceptable as they do not allow proper verification of the data in CRFs. Also, it is important to review the whole record to determine whether there is any conflict with CRF entries.

To ensure direct access, the study subject consent form must clearly indicate that permission for access has been granted by the study subject. Similarly, the investigator agreement must state that direct access is required and accepted. Special arrangements with medical records departments in hospitals or clinics may be required and this should be determined in the early stages of setting up the study. To respect confidentiality, the monitor will not remove confidential documents from the study site (e.g. take documents to a hotel room) to conduct source data verification. The monitor will not photocopy documents with study subject names: if it is necessary to photocopy documents, these must be anonymised before removal from the study site.

It is unethical to conduct a study without direct access to source documents and the ensuing source data verification procedure. First, if data are not verified, they may be dangerous – we know from experience that unless source data verification is undertaken, there will be many data errors. Second, the regulators (certainly the FDA) will insist on direct access – if this is not granted, the study will be rejected. Thus, the study will have been conducted for no purpose and the study subjects will have been exposed to risk for no valid reason.

A review of our audit database indicated that there was no access (or significantly restricted access) to source documents, or there were no source documents, at 12% of 378 sites. In the USA, where the regulators have required access to source documents for many years, it has been well understood by the pharmaceutical industry and investigators that direct access is necessary. In some other countries, where inspection has barely begun, the necessity for direct access is still not fully accepted. In countries such as the UK, there are still local ethics committees and hospital administrations which are resistant to direct access, and there are still sponsors/CROs which will actually allow a study to begin under those conditions. Some individuals, particularly sponsor/CRO personnel, have tried to explain this situation by arguing that access to clinical notes is 'illegal' in some countries. We have never actually seen regulatory documentation to support this rationale.

... A study of back pain, UK, 25 patients
The investigator agreed to direct access to source documents by the FDA (if they were to inspect), but did not allow direct access for the monitor or the auditor. He signed the CRFs, indicating that he had himself done the source data review. He kept cards with study data separate from normal medical notes and explained that he did not wish to clutter the original records. It is almost guaranteed, based on experience, that if source document verification is not undertaken by the monitor, data quality will not be good. Thus, even though this investigator would have allowed access to the inspectors, the study would have probably failed the inspection.

... A study of hypertension, UK, 43 patients
There was no access to source documents and the investigator had written to the sponsor that this was a restriction imposed by the ethics committee. The auditors asked him to provide evidence of this restriction and he finally admitted that it was actually a restriction imposed by himself, not the ethics committee.

... A study of allergies, Germany, 14 patients
During the audit, the monitor turned on the investigator's computer, entered the password and was able to peruse information as she wished. Information on all patients at the clinic (not just the study subjects) were available to the monitor. To assure site personnel and study subjects that confidentiality will be fully respected, this situation should never occur. Monitors should only be permitted to observe the source documents for the enrolled study subjects.

... A study of an anticoagulant, Italy, 10 patients
The on-line computer system for randomisation required the investigator to provide the full study subject name to the CRO prior to issue of treatment allocation. Confidential names were thus maintained on the database of the CRO. Sponsors and CROs must never have full study subject names on any documentation maintained on their premises.

5.3   SOURCE DATA VERIFICATION

Source data verification is the process of verifying CRF entries against data in the source documents. Source data verification is only carried out at the study site, usually by the sponsor/ CRO monitor. (Auditors will also conduct source data verification on a sample of CRFs. Inspectors may conduct source data verification on a sample or all CRFs.)

The extent of source data verification should be documented by the monitor on a special source data verification form which must be attached to the relevant monitor reports. A customised source data verification form should be prepared for each study and the monitor must record all deviations or discrepancies in data on this form, unless the deviations or discrepancies are resolved at the time of the monitoring visit. The monitor must inform all site personnel of discrepancies so that procedures can be improved in future.

Source data verification will be most intense at the beginning of the study and whenever new subjects are entered. The monitor must allow adequate time for this activity. Thereafter, at subsequent monitoring visits, the monitor must check all new data entered in source documents. With some studies it is not unusual for the monitor to require a half day for one study subject. Checklists 5.3–1 and 5.3–2 provide details on the data items which require review by the monitor. Some data (to be decided and documented in advance) may be checked on a sampling basis. If significant errors are detected, a complete check may be required. The acceptable error rate should be established before data review.

. . . The SOPs of the UK subsidiary of a large multinational pharmaceutical company.
In the top margin of the sponsor's SOP for source data verification was a small handwritten note which stated 'we hardly ever do this'!

How much information is expected in source documents? This is a difficult issue, but one that must be discussed and resolved before the CRFs are completed. In fact, we recommend the investigators do not sign protocols until the source data requirements have been fully explained to them.

Source documents did not clearly indicate study participation at 51% of 378 sites in our audit database. Often, there was a cryptic entry (e.g. 'Study 123' or 'Company X Study') which would not have provided adequate information for healthcare workers who might be responsible for the patient in the future. The cause for this finding is usually poor record-keeping by study site personnel and lack of careful oversight by monitors. In some countries (e.g. Germany), there was a deliberate attempt to ensure that the clinical notes did not show that patients were in pharmaceutical industry-sponsored research for fear of how this might be reviewed by the insurance companies and how costs would also be allocated. This sometimes led to the preparation of two sets of notes, one for normal clinical care and one for the purposes of the study. The auditors were very concerned with this procedure as the two sets might differ, and it would be difficult for the monitors and auditors to be sure a full and complete set of notes was being reviewed. It is important that other treating physicians are aware that the patient was, or is, in a clinical study.

Further, source documents did not clearly describe exposure to the study treatment (e.g. start and stop dates of treatment, changes in dosing, missed doses, etc.) at 54% of 378 sites and visit dates were not confirmed in the source documents at 32% of those sites. Again, it is important that other treating physicians are fully aware of the details of exposure to study treatments.

... A Phase I study, UK, 12 healthy volunteers
The investigator reported that recording 'back pain' in the source documents was a general term used when individuals required time off work to be in studies.

... A study of cardiovascular surgery, Belgium, 101 patients
To indicate participation in the study, the clinical notes indicated 'pump on': the investigator explained that a clearer entry would have caused problems with insurance companies. Clinical notes are prepared for patients, not insurance companies or pharmaceutical companies. It is important that the records contain all information necessary to take care of the patients.

The primary care physician (family doctor or general practitioner or referring physician) was not notified of study participation at 57% of 378 sites in our audit database. The poor compliance for this item ranged from 41% (UK) to 79% (USA). The relatively better performance in the UK was probably due to the strong referral system among physicians: most patients are registered with a general practitioner who might refer them to consultants for specialist care. The relatively worse performance in the USA was probably linked to the fact that many patients do not have a primary care physician and turn up for specialist care as they wish (and as they can afford!). Informing a primary care physician of study participation can be a very important point in confirming eligibility, particularly in study subjects that present de novo or respond to advertisements. It is often argued that in countries such as the USA, Germany and France, it is not possible to confirm entry criteria with primary care physicians, but most subjects presenting for clinical studies have previously been seen by another physician who could verify some information. There is a precedent for establishing primary care physician contact as normal procedure for Phase I studies to confirm the history of healthy volunteers and ensure that they are not entering studies concurrently or too often. Otherwise, sponsors and CROs do not seem to press compliance with this item and basically defer to the wishes of local investigators and ethics committees. In the UK, many ethics committees do require contact with primary care physicians, but this is apparently ignored.

... A Phase I study, Eire, nine healthy volunteers
There was no notification of family doctors. The investigator explained that the study subjects were all students or physicians who were not registered with a family doctor. There was no other evidence of confirmation of medical history.

In our audit database, source documents did not support (provided no evidence or inadequate evidence) the selection of suitable study subjects at 30% of 378 sites. The poor level of compliance basically implied that inappropriate subjects were being entered in clinical studies. The tremendous pressure to recruit as quickly as possible probably contributed to a lack of rigour in recruitment criteria. (After each monitoring visit, the monitor will be asked by managers – how many patients are in the study? In turn, the monitors will immediately telephone the study sites and ask – where are the patients?) Poor monitoring, caused by poor standards set by the companies employing the monitors, was probably the most important contributing factor to non-compliance. Some of the problems related to ensuring that information in source documents was correctly transcribed into CRFs: this is a primary monitoring role. Other problems related to ensuring that clinical notes were adequately comprehensive and supportive of inclusion and exclusion criteria. Some national differences in record-keeping might have a small role in non-compliance. Record-keeping standards, for clinical notes, were similar in most countries: notes were often meagre and illegible. (However, our auditors have often commented on the relatively better record-keeping in countries such as the Czech Republic, Hungary, Poland and the United Arab Emirates. There was usually more attention to detail in those notes.) Nevertheless, even with excellent source documents, compliance will be poor if monitoring is inadequate.

Lack of evidence of selection criteria was especially prevalent in studies with referred study subjects or subjects recruited by advertisement. This was particularly troublesome in some therapeutic areas: (e.g. hormone replacement therapy, headache studies, 'tummy upset' studies). Study subjects in these cases were entered *de novo* (previously unknown to the investigator) and the clinical basis (as evidenced by information in the source documents) upon which the decision was made to enter such individuals into clinical studies was not obvious. It would appear that many investigators allow individuals into studies without much prior clinical knowledge of them. The auditors were especially concerned about this problem in the USA, where the situation was possibly exacerbated by the fact that patients were often attracted to clinical studies as the only means to afford treatment.

. . . A study of an anxiolytic, UK, 13 patients
In seven subjects, there was no evidence of generalised anxiety disorder in the source documents.

. . . A study of hypertension, UK, 28 patients.
Some patients in the study did not actually belong to the practice of the

investigator. He had no direct knowledge of these patients, but he had signed the CRFs for all of them. Investigator signatures on CRFs are usually required to confirm the reliability of the data in the CRFs.

... A study of hormone replacement therapy, France, 19 study subjects
As soon as study subjects entered the study, the investigator stopped recording any information in their normal medical notes, only in CRFs. Investigators must be taught that CRF entries do not substitute for source documents, with few exceptions.

The quality of source documents is extremely important – these documents must last for many years.

... A study of hypertension, UK, 33 patients
The ECG traces and 24-hour blood pressure printouts were recorded on heat-sensitive paper: they were fading by the time of the audit, only a few months after completion of the study. This is a common finding in studies which use thermal paper for printouts of data.

... A study of a diagnostic agent, Germany, four patients
The auditors found that the paper printouts of laboratory test results were very neatly cut so that they could be pasted into the small space allocated in the patient's clinical notes. The names and dates associated with the test results were cut off! Many study sites are not meticulous with ensuring that credible identifiers are included on source documents. In many clinical records, we find bits of paper with no name, date or identification of the individual responsible for the data entry. The best notes we observed were in an oncology facility in Hungary: patient records were maintained in bound notebooks, all pages were numbered consecutively and all entries were in chronological order, and each entry was initialled and dated. Many notes were written in Hungarian and Latin!

... A study of an anxiolytic, France, 12 patients
The investigator could not read his own writing – nor could anyone else. Any experienced monitor will confirm that this is a serious problem. If the handwriting is illegible, the notes are useless. Sponsor/CROs may need to insist on supplemental typed copies of notes, signed and dated and prepared by the site

personnel. (The original illegible notes should never be discarded.)

Checklist 5.3–1. Initial Monitor Review and Retrieval of CRFs at the Investigator Site

The sponsor/CRO monitor will review the following CRF items at study sites:

- All entries on to CRFs must be legible. If the handwriting is not legible, a data query must be issued, completed by the site personnel and signed by the investigator. The 'illegible' copy must be retained.

- All entries on original CRFs must be made in ink. Pencilled entries are not acceptable as they may be modified without leaving evidence of the modification.

- A list must be maintained of all individuals permitted to make entries in original CRFs. The sponsor/CRO personnel may never make entries on the top (white original) copies of CRFs or on the copies left at the investigator site except in clearly designated areas.

- Corrections must be made by crossing through the incorrect entry and putting the correct information by its side. The incorrect entry must remain visible and the correction must be initialled and dated by the investigator (or authorised delegate) making the correction. A reason should be documented for all changes. (There will be lots of argument on this point. Many people will argue that the reason is obvious. This is usually not the case. See some of our stories. Make it simple – produce a code list for reasons.) The correction must be legible on all copies of the CRF page.

- Blank CRF pages (e.g. missed visits, early terminations, extra forms) must also be collected by the monitor.

- Extra documents to be attached to CRFs (and which will be archived by the sponsor/CRO) must be anonymised before retrieval. Such documents might include diagnostic reports for eligibility, ECGs, ECHOs, MUGAs, autopsy report, laboratory reports, etc. The types of extra documents to be collected must be determined in advance to ensure no errors in protecting subject confidentiality.

- Before retrieval, all collected CRFs must be signed by the investigator to indicate that the data are correct and accurate to the best of the investigator's knowledge. CRFs may never be collected without the investigator's authorisation; therefore, unless individual CRF pages require investigator signatures, it is only possible to retrieve complete sections or modules of CRFs at any particular visit.

Checklist 5.3–2. Extent of Source Data Verification

For all study subjects, source data verification will proceed with a review of data for the following items:

- Existence of medical records/files at the study site. There must be a medical file, separate from the CRF, which forms a normal part of the record for the study subjects. The medical file should clearly indicate the full name, birth date and hospital/clinic/health service number of the study subject.
- Eligibility of study subjects (compliance with inclusion/exclusion criteria). The medical file must show compliance with the inclusion and exclusion criteria. As it is rare that a medical file will support all evidence (with regard to the selection of study subjects) required in a clinical study CRF, considerable judgement is needed in assessing this item. At a minimum, demographic characteristics (e.g. sex, weight and height), diagnoses (e.g. major condition for which the subject was being treated) and other 'hard' data (e.g. laboratory results within a specified range or normal chest x-ray) should be clearly indicated in the medical files. Absence of 'positive evidence' of an exclusion criterion may be acceptable, but this must be considered carefully. If the medical file has little or no information of medical history, it would not support selection of the subject. All required baseline assessments must be evident.
- Indication of participation in the study. The medical file should clearly show that the subject was in a clinical study. A code or study number alone is not adequate. For the protection of the study subject, the record should note participation in case the information is necessary for future clinical care. The notation might be as follows: 'Entered study (number, medication/device, sponsor/CRO name) on [date]. Consent obtained. Study medication administered on [date].'
- Consent procedures. The original signed consent form should be maintained with the subject's medical files or in the investigator files, if not permitted by the hospital or clinical setting. Otherwise, an indication that consent was obtained (with the date specified)

should be noted in the medical files. Signatures and date must be checked carefully to ensure that the correct individuals were involved in the consent procedure and that consent was obtained prior to any study intervention. If a revised consent form was used, both the original and the revised form must be in the source documents.

- Record of exposure to study medication/device. The medical file should clearly indicate when treatment began, when treatment finished, and all intervening treatment dates. The dispensing records, which are normally separate from the medical file, must also be examined to determine exposure to study medication/device.

- Record of concomitant medications/devices. All notations of previous and concomitant medication/device use must be examined. All entries in the CRF should be verifiable in the medical file by name, date(s) of administration, dose and reason (or indication). All entries in the medical file during the time period specified by the protocol must be noted in the CRF. Concomitant medication/device use must be explicable by an appropriate indication. They must be consistent from visit to visit. The reasons (indications) for use of concomitant medications/devices, newly prescribed during the study period, must be noted as AEs. The medical history should be reviewed to determine whether medical conditions arising during the study already existed at baseline.

- Visit dates. All visit dates should be recorded in the medical file. Interim visit dates recorded in the medical file, but not in the CRF, should be noted by the monitor in case they signify occurrence of AEs or protocol violations. The final visit date should be so indicated (e.g. 'study finished' or 'withdrew from study').

- AEs. All AEs noted in the medical file during the time period specified by the protocol must be recorded in the CRF. Normally, all AEs recorded in the CRF should also be recorded in the medical file. In some studies, it may be acceptable that minor expected events are only recorded in the CRF, but this must be considered on a case-by-case basis. The monitor must also carefully check other documents (e.g. diary cards, quality of life forms) for sources of information about AEs. Occurrence of out-of-range laboratory values, which are considered to be clinically significant by the investigator, must be reported and assessed as AEs.

- Major safety and efficacy variables (to be decided and documented in advance). It is not necessary for all measured variables to be recorded in the medical file. Present and future clinical care of the study subject is the most important factor in determining whether or not measured variables should be recorded in the medical file. The investigator should record what he/she would normally record to care for the study subject, but also take into account any recording needed because of the special circumstances of a clinical study. The medical file should be reviewed entirely to ensure that no additional information exists in the medical file which should have been recorded in the CRF.

5.4 DATA QUERIES

Although the monitor will spend considerable time checking all data at the study site, it is not possible to do this task perfectly. The monitor is usually focused on one patient at a time, but many types of data errors do not show up until a comparison is made across study subjects. The complexities of the data trail (e.g. from source documents to CRFs to computer listing to data display to final reports) offer many opportunities to introduce error. We must do our best to minimise the error.

There is only one way to avoid handling data queries – do not do clinical research. Issue of data queries is a normal process: investigators and monitors should worry if no data queries are issued as this probably indicates a lack of careful scrutiny of the data. Monitors become as 'annoyed' as investigators with data queries – probably because the monitors must follow through with the queries. Many feel the data processing personnel ask 'picky' 'non-relevant' questions. But no one should resist this process – the queries are normally quite legitimate and worthwhile. Data processing personnel are taught to look at data in a different fashion – their review is critical to ensuring good data. Inevitably this further review will result in further questions about the data and this will result in the issue of data queries. (Incidentally data processing personnel should try to resist labelling monitors and site personnel as 'sloppy' – clinical data are notoriously subjective and sometimes vague – but the data personnel must persist in demanding the best possible data. All sides need to co-operate in this process.)

In our audit database, there were significant discrepancies between the data in source documents and the data in CRFs at 41% of 378 sites. Further, there were discrepancies between laboratory reports and CRF data at 54% of the sites and discrepancies between main effectiveness variables recorded in CRFs compared to source medical records at 50% of the sites. This is certainly the 'number one' reason why studies might fail in the eyes of the FDA. Poor monitoring, again attributed to varying sponsor/CRO standards, is the most important factor in noncompliance with this item. Quality of source documents is also a contributing factor. Many sponsors and CROs also experience problems in countries with computerised data due to the lack of security of the data and the lack of an audit trail in the electronic system. If it cannot be determined when data were entered, and by whom, are the data credible?

Further review, verification and clarification of data, after CRFs have been returned to the sponsor/CRO must be undertaken carefully. The initial internal review may require that the CRFs will be reviewed by a second monitor (i.e. secondary monitoring) before delivery to the data processing personnel (Checklist 5.4–1). A record must be maintained of all CRFs retrieved and processed. CRFs must be reviewed by all responsible reviewers in the clinical research department within a specified time period (e.g. five working days) of retrieval from the investigator site. The sponsor/CRO must not make any entries on original top copies of retrieved CRFs or on copies of CRFs at the investigator site. Also, data recorded on CRFs should be entered into the computer as quickly as possible (e.g. within 10 working days of being received by the data processing group). After the data are entered into the computer, any questions concerning the data should be sent to the monitor who will, if necessary, contact the investigator for resolution of the data.

After the CRFs have been reviewed by the monitor at the investigator site, signed by the investigator and brought back to the sponsor/CRO, the data contained within these CRFs cannot be changed except by means of a formal data clarification and resolution procedure, as described below. All data changes must be authorised by the investigator ultimately. Obviously, the sponsor/CRO cannot arbitrarily make changes of data. In our audit database, data changes (in CRFs or data query/resolution forms) were not approved (initialled and dated) by an authorised person at the study site at 41% of 378 sites.

Requests for data clarification and resolution must be documented on a data query form, which must be issued quickly (e.g. within five working days of retrieval of the CRF to the sponsor/ CRO premises). The data query form will be printed on three-part paper, with completed copies ultimately designated for: the sponsor/CRO archives (original copy); investigator CRF archives (bottom copy) and data processing personnel (usually the middle copy). (The source data verification form must be distinguished from the date query form. The former is prepared at the study site during the monitoring visit and discrepancies are resolved as they arise: the data query form is issued after CRFs have been retrieved by the sponsor/CRO and the duplicate pages of the CRFs have been separated by the monitor at the study site.)

The data query form must be handled like an extension to the CRF and treated with the same care. The original form should be taken by the monitor to the study site for completion and signature by the investigator, and for source data verification. (If sent by post, the monitor must subsequently visit the study site to verify the data resolution.) After completion and signature by the investigator, the bottom copy of the data query form should be retained with the investigator copy of the CRF. The original and middle copy are usually returned to the sponsor/CRO. The original copy of the data query form will immediately be archived, with the original relevant CRF pages: the second copy will be forwarded for use by data entry and processing personnel. Data entry on the computer by the sponsor/CRO might occur before an investigator signature is obtained on the data query form. However, the database cannot be 'locked' until all signed data query forms are received and verified.

... A study of the pharmacokinetics of a drug administered during anaesthesia, France, 97 patients
Patients were required to meet a specified height-weight ratio. For some patients, the original height (which made the patient ineligible) was changed to make the patient eligible. One patient's height apparently increased by 8 centimetres. The investigator could not explain these changes. The monitor must insist on written explanations for data changes such as these.

... A study of a prostaglandin, Germany, 40 patients
The study required a six-hour continuous infusion every day for 28 days. The CRFs indicated that the infusion started at exactly 09.15 hours for all patients. The investigator was adamant that this was correct. The auditors were not convinced that this was possible and further investigation of the nursing notes indicated that the infusions started between 01.00 and 02.00 hours at much more credible intervals. It is easier for reviewers who have access to several patients' data to observe such patterns than it is for the monitor who is normally focused on one patient at a time.

... A study of an anxiolytic, France, eight patients
The psychiatric rating scales were changed several weeks after the original assessment. The changes made patients who were previously ineligible become eligible. The auditors queried the changes, but no explanations were provided. These kinds of events will definitely arouse questions about the honesty of the data.

... A study of an anxiolytic, France, 15 patients
There were several new entries in CRFs which were recorded up to four months after the original entries on the medical history page. Apparently the information was subsequently provided to the investigator by the patients. It is important to collect data as soon as they are observed or reported. 'Old' data quickly lose credibility.

Checklist 5.4–1. Initial Internal CRF Review

The following questions will be addressed during the initial CRF review at the sponsor/CRO premises:

- Is the study subject eligible? The protocol violations affecting eligibility should be specified.
- Is the study subject evaluable for safety? The protocol violations affecting safety evaluability should be specified.
- Is the study subject evaluable for effectiveness? The protocol violations affecting effectiveness evaluability should be specified.
- Did the study subject complete the study? If not, the reasons for premature termination and the impact on evaluability should be specified.
- Were AEs noted? If yes, the medical adviser should be notified

promptly (e.g. within two working days). The AEs should be specified.
- Were SAEs noted? If yes, the medical adviser should be notified immediately. The SAEs should be specified.
- Did the subject withdraw due to AEs? The AEs resulting in withdrawal should be specified.
- Did the subjects withdraw due to ineffectiveness of the study medication/device? If yes, the events should be specified.
- Is the study subject a dropout?
- Is data resolution required? If yes, a data query form should be attached and issued.

5.5   GENERAL INTERNAL DATA PROCESSING

Eventually, after resolution of all data queries, the data management department will produce data listings and other presentations of data (e.g. tables, graphs, figures) which should be reviewed by the monitor. Any new queries or errors detected during review of the data presentation must be sent to the data entry personnel. As a result of the review of the data listings, the monitor or data processing personnel may decide that further data queries must be issued to the investigator.

'Data conventions' refer to the variations to protocol requirements which will be permitted for statistical analysis. The data conventions will normally be determined during the development of the protocol. Further refinement of the definition of data conventions may arise during the performance of the study. All proposed data conventions are to be discussed and agreed in a formal meeting which should be documented. Final data conventions will be established and documented before the statistical analysis of the study.

'Subject classification' refers to the final determination of eligibility and evaluability of study subjects within the limits of the data conventions. Final determination of subject classification requires the assistance of the monitor and other clinical research personnel, and the biostatistician must also approve all final decisions. Data listings, blinded to treatment allocation, of all exceptions to the data conventions and copies of the agreed data conventions form will be issued prior to final decisions about subject classification. Subject classification will be determined and documented after clinical completion of the study, but prior to unblinding (in the case of a double-blind study). After data clarification and resolution has been completed and just prior to statistical analysis, all issues relating to inclusion/ exclusion of subjects for analysis must be resolved to enable formal subject classification to be achieved.

For each subject, if a protocol variation falls within the limits of the data conventions, the subject may be considered to be eligible for determination of evaluability. An assessment of whether the subject is evaluable, within the bounds of the data conventions, must also be made. A meeting will be held to determine which variations to the protocol will be considered acceptable in deciding the eligibility and evaluability of subjects to be included in the assessment of the safety and efficacy of the study medication/device. If the protocol variation is a violation of the data conventions, the subjects will be assessed on a subject-by-subject basis for eligibility and evaluability. A final blinded subject classification document listing acceptability for safety and efficacy analyses will be prepared and documented after all questions regarding protocol variations have been resolved.

It is critical that all data review procedures described in this chapter be prompt. As time goes by, it becomes more and more difficult to correct data. Slow processing means that data resolution loses credibility.

. . . A study of prostate cancer, UK, 36 patients
Data processing started between one and two years after completion of subjects in the study. This is a common occurrence at many study sites due to changing priorities in a busy clinical research department. Many types of data simply cannot be resolved after such a lengthy time period. All studies must come to completion – it is unethical to treat patients in studies which are left to 'languish' indefinitely.

5.6   GENERAL STATISTICAL PROCEDURES

Expert advice is needed to deal with statistical issues, and this section is only intended to highlight a few points which might be of importance to monitors and study site personnel.

A statistical analysis plan must be prepared before a clinical study begins. This requires the input of a properly qualified biostatistician. Similarly, a proper statistical analysis should be conducted and reported at the end of each clinical study. The statistical analysis plan for a clinical study will be written by the biostatistician responsible for the analysis of the study in consultation with the clinical team. The statistical analysis plan must be written and approved by the sponsor/ CRO prior to the issue of the final approved protocol. Approval of the statistical analysis plan must be documented. A synopsis of the statistical analysis plan should be included in the protocol. (Thus, it is available for external review by ethics committees and regulators.)

The statistical analysis of a study may only commence after the study has been completed and the data are 'clean'. When the database has been declared to be 'clean' and has been formally 'locked' (that is, no further changes can be made to the database), final statistical analysis may be performed according to the statistical plan. The database must be formally locked by authorisation from a designated individual and at that time further access to the data in the database will be denied. The monitor and other clinical research personnel must be informed of the locking procedure. The database will then be formally released to the biostatistician for the final statistical analysis. Any exceptions (i.e. interim analyses) must be documented with reasons. The biostatistician must be provided with a subject-by-subject listing to specify in which analyses each subject may be included (e.g. intent-to-treat, valid case analysis, special case, etc.). In the case of blind studies, the randomisation schedule will be released to the biostatistician after the statistical analyses have been completed in order that assignment of treatments to the study groups can be completed.

After the final statistical report has been completed it will be issued with the signed approval of the biostatistician. The approval of the biostatistician implies that: all data have been included in the analysis and any exclusions have been clearly stated in the report; data have been accurately tabulated and summarised; all listings, tables and graphs in the report are correct; and statistical methodology is correct.

CASE STUDY FIVE

A Multi-Centre Double-Blind Study to Assess the Analgesic Activity of Drug X Compared with Placebo in Approximately 200 Patients with Osteoarthritis (Europe).

The auditors were asked to assess this completed study because of the finding, after independent statistical review, of opposite results in the two study sites: at one site, drug A was better than placebo and at the other site, placebo was better than drug A. This is a nightmarish situation for any company and needs explanation. The CRO claimed to have conducted full source data verification, but the auditors found the data to be completely unreliable at both study sites. Some of the individual data errors were minor (and occur in all studies we have audited), but given that numerous errors were observed in almost all patients in this study, overall credibility of data was lost. The study was eventually abandoned. More than 200 patients were treated for nothing!

Unless otherwise indicated, the problems noted below related to both study sites, referred to as Sites A (more than 60 subjects) and B (more than 140 subjects). 'Site' B in fact was a co-ordinating centre for at least 30 other contributing sites, involving more than 40 general practitioners.

The main effectiveness endpoint for this study was the patient's self-assessment using a visual analogue scale (VAS). Patients were instructed to indicate their pain intensity on a 10 centimetre line – 0 centimetre for no pain and 10 centimetres for severe pain. To be eligible for the study, baseline pain had to be at least 5 centimetres in intensity.

Summary of Major Deficiencies

Standard Operating Procedures: Many important SOP topics were not addressed (e.g. training/qualifications of CRO personnel; investigator brochures; selection of clinical laboratories; financial payments to investigators and study subjects; data management; statistical procedures; randomisation procedures; and study medication requisition, packaging, labelling, shipment, control at the study site and final disposition/destruction).

Ethics Committee Review: The date and version number of the protocol submitted to the ethics committees for review and approval were not clearly stated in the letters of approval, which did not specify the documents reviewed. Several required items were apparently not assessed by the ethics committees before the study began. There was no evidence to suggest any further review at either site during and after the study.

At Site B, the ethics committee was apparently only informed of two of the participating investigators: there were actually more than 40 physicians assessing patients. (The sponsor was unaware of this finding until the audit was undertaken.) The committee had requested a change in the consent form to ensure that access to source documents was clearly described to study subjects: this change was not made on all consent forms. The ethics committee which made the decision for this study apparently included only four members. Since one member was an investigator (he declared a conflict of interest), only three members apparently made the decision concerning this study. (It is unlikely that this small number provided adequate representation for a safe ethics committee approval.)

Informed Consent Procedures: Several important items of information were not provided to study subjects. At Site B, the fact that confidential records would be reviewed by the sponsor or CRO personnel and regulatory authorities was not consistently stated on all copies of the consent form, although the ethics committee had requested this change. Some subjects signed consent forms where this requirement was not clearly stated.

At Site A, there were some irregularities in the consent procedure: the dates were rarely recorded by the study subject themselves, but were usually recorded by the investigator; there was no provision on the consent form for the investigator to separately sign and print his name and write the date; and the obtaining of consent was not documented for any study subjects by the signature of a witness.

At Site B, there were also irregularities in the consent procedure: for at least four subjects, it appeared that the study nurse had signed the subjects' names in the place of the subject – the same nurse was involved in all observed cases.; one subject had crossed out the sentence allowing direct access to source documents; dates were rarely recorded by the study subjects themselves, but were usually recorded by the study nurse or an 'investigator' (physician); in at least 11 cases, the consent forms were signed by physicians who were not responsible for the source documents for those subjects, further confusing determination of who was actually responsible for the subjects in the study; names of the physicians providing information to study subjects were not recorded on the consent forms for at least six subjects; original signed consent forms were not usually available at the individual contributing investigator sites – they were retained at the main co-ordinating site; there was no provision on the consent forms for the investigator to separately sign and print his/her name and write the date; the dates of consent form signatures were not apparently recorded by the investigators, but were recorded by the witness (who was usually a study nurse); and although the obtaining of consent was documented for all study subjects by the signature of a witness, the witness was apparently one of the study nurses and in some cases, the investigator signed as the witness.

At both sites, for some subjects, X-rays had been performed just prior to the screening visit and the obtaining of consent. The auditors considered it likely that these X-rays were performed for the purpose of inclusion into the study prior to the obtaining of consent.

Protocol: At Site A, some protocol signatures were not obtained until after more than 50 study subjects had received treatment. At Site B, only one physician signed the protocol as the investigator –

he was responsible for only three subjects enrolled at this site. No other 'investigators' had signed the protocol. At least 40 different physicians were involved in obtaining consent, conducting the pre-study and post-study physical examination and preparing source documents. Some protocol signatures were not obtained until after all subjects had been recruited to the study.

The protocol was missing many important items. In particular, the sections on study subject selection, study medications, AEs, randomization procedures, monitoring, data handling and statistical analysis and ethical considerations lacked necessary information.

There was no evidence that the protocol amendment was reviewed/approved by the ethics committee or regulatory authority. At both sites, some signatures on the protocol amendment were obtained after the study had closed. At Site B, only one of the more than 40 participating physicians had signed the protocol amendment.

CRF Design: There were significant deficiencies in the CRF design for the following data collection requirements: details of previous medications and therapies; details of compliance with the use of the study medication by the study subject; and details of AEs.

Setting Up the Study: There were no instructions in the investigator brochure (or any other document) for handling of the study medication. At Site B, there was no evidence that the brochure had been distributed to each of the more than 40 'investigators' contributing to the study.

In the statements of qualifications of investigators, there was usually no indication of whether they had other clinical research commitments or whether the investigators had adequate time for the study. At Site B, there were no CVs for at least six physicians who had been involved in the informed consent process and declared as investigators on the consent forms. CVs for approximately 70 general practitioners and 10 study nurses were in the study files. The physicians were distributed among at least 30 different locations. (At least 40 different physicians were involved in obtaining consent, conducting the pre-study and post-study physical examination and preparing source documents.)

There was no evidence of a pre-study site assessment report at either site. At Site A, the initiation visit documentation was dated after the first patient started treatment. At Site B, the initiation visit, held only at the co-ordinating centre, was attended by one physician and a study nurse. There were no other formal initiation visits.

Monitoring: At both sites, the monitor reports did not document several important topics. In particular, the reports did not document the general quality of the CRFs, correct reporting of AEs, the handling of study medication and compliance of use of medication by study subjects. Study closure was not sufficiently documented. At Site B, there was no evidence that the monitor had checked source documents at each of the contributing investigator sites as the monitor reports only indicated that the co-ordinating centre had been visited. Apparently a 'summary document', prepared by the CRO, was considered to be the source document. (The auditors did not accept this as a valid source document.)

Control of Clinical Study Medication: The study file did not contain information about movement of study medication from the sponsor to the CRO and the management of medication on the CRO premises. The information on the shipment notes from the CRO to the study sites, and on the receipt notes, was inadequate and many details were missing (e.g. pharmacist address, shipment date, date of shipment letter, method of shipment, handling instructions, storage instructions, description of items shipped, dose strength, quantity per package, number of packages, batch numbers, and expiry date). At Site B the acknowledgement of receipt forms were signed by two individuals who were not identified in the study file. There was no confirmation that storage conditions were met after receipt, that at the time of receipt supplies were within the limits of the expiry date and that the supplies were received in good order. One shipment of study medication apparently took seven to eight days to be delivered; there was no documentation of the conditions during shipment.

The documentation of storage of study medication at both study sites was inadequate. The investigators were not required to maintain a log of the temperature for the medication storage area. At Site A, the medication was stored in an attic without a lock on the door. The medication was almost certain to have been subject to fluctuating environmental temperatures. There was no temperature-control device in place and a record of daily temperatures was not taken. At Site B, there was no documentation of maintenance of temperature in the medication storage area and there was no documentation of storage of medication at any of the other contributing sites. Personnel at site B reported that the medication was immediately given to the study subjects by study nurses when the nurses visited the individual study sites, but this was not adequately documented. There was no record of how long medications were retained by study nurses during transit, usually by car. Dispensing records were inadequate and medication had not been dispensed in the correct sequence. At Site B, the dispensing record did not indicate the contributing sites to which the medication had been taken.

There was inadequate evidence of assessment of compliance with use of the study medication and there were problems in compliance with use of study medication, as evidenced by the measured amount of medication remaining in the containers. Even though study subjects were provided with a device for measuring the correct amount of medication to apply, the total amount that had been used by each subject by the end of the study varied so that it appeared that many of the subjects had not complied with correct use of the study medication. In a letter, a CRO staff member implied that compliance had been affected by 'how liquid the medication was' (probably because of the overly warm storage conditions). The final return and disposition of study medication was inadequately recorded. Neither the CRO nor the investigators were provided with emergency randomisation codebreak envelopes during the study, although this was a double-blind study.

Filing/Archiving: Files at the CRO and investigator sites were not adequately secure and fire resistant. At the CRO, the files/archives were kept in a locked cupboard but in an open room without a door. Different types of documents were retained in one box without indexing. Some important items were not present in the CRO and investigator files. Copies of audit reports were noted in the CRO files. (Audit reports should be filed separately.) At Site A the files/archives were kept in an unlocked attic cupboard. At Site B, there was no evidence that the monitor had checked the security of source documents at each of the contributing investigator sites. (At one contributing centre the auditors were shown to the treatment room, but no site personnel were present. The source documents had been placed on the examining bed. Medications and documents for another study were in an unlocked open cabinet, available to anyone in the room.)

Source Data – Site A: With regard to availability of source documents, only photocopies of parts of the source medical records were evident for some subjects: full medical records were either at a different practice or were moved with subjects who had gone to other practices. Copies of these records did not always include the visit dates to which the notes pertained. Handwriting in the source medical records was not always legible. Parts of the source documents (in particular, concomitant medication information) consisted of data in electronic format. A signed and dated printout of those data was not available.

Owing to limited information on eligibility entered in the source medical records, the auditors could not assess eligibility for all study subjects. Frequently, X-rays had not been performed or reports were not available at the time the subject was entered into the study, as judged from the dates on the X-ray reports. There was no evidence in the source documents to support information about the physical examination, vital signs and weight and height. Many other subjects were recruited to the study who did not meet the inclusion criteria stated in the protocol and there were several discrepancies in baseline data. Examples included:

12 subjects: No X-ray – primary diagnosis not confirmed.

10 subjects: Source documents indicated other conditions prohibited by protocol – protocol violations.

5 subjects: The baseline VAS score was below 5 centimetres – protocol violations.

4 subjects: Subject's X-ray performed more than six months before study–protocol violations.

4 subjects: According to X-ray, primary diagnosis not confirmed.

3 subjects: Source documents indicated sensitivity to analgesic drugs – protocol violations.

3 subjects: Source documents indicated concurrent use of prohibited analgesics – protocol violations.

The medical history as noted in the source medical records had not been adequately described in the CRF for more than 40 study subjects. Discrepancies in the use of concomitant medication were noted in a comparison of the source medical records and the CRFs in more than 30 patients. Not all medication taken in the last three months prior to the study and during the study (required to be recorded according to the protocol), as indicated on the investigators' computerised database, had been entered in the CRF. Discrepancies in AE reporting were noted between the source medical records and the CRFs in 15 patients.

The main effectiveness variables (pain rating) were recorded in the CRF and the diary cards. There were no details in the source medical records to verify efficacy data. Sometimes CRFs were completed by different investigators for the same patient and the comparability of investigator scores could be questioned. Completion of the VAS was not always correct. For many patients, crosses were used to mark the VAS score, which either did not cross the VAS lines at all or crossed it twice. VAS rating scales completed by study subjects had been corrected by the investigators for eight subjects. For example, pain was modified by the investigator from a value <5 cm (which would exclude the subject from participation in the study) to a value >5 cm (subject could be included). The reason given by the investigator was that the subject misunderstood the instructions (or no reason was provided). The auditors considered this of great importance as the corrections changed the eligibility of study subjects.

Source Data – Site B: Photocopies of CRFs (and diary cards) for the audit sample were not obtained prior to the audit due to time constraints. The auditors were not aware, at the time of the CRO audit, that subjects at this centre were actually treated at several different locations. The designated investigator who had signed the protocol, had only been responsible for three study subjects. Therefore, the actual sites to be audited were not determined until a few days before the audit. At least 40 different physicians were involved in obtaining consent, conducting the pre-study and post-study physical examination and preparing source documents.

The source records did not provide adequate evidence that all study subjects met the selection criteria specified in the protocol. Apart from the information entered on the 'summary documents' (basic demographics, medical history, physical examination, vital signs, weight and height, the extent of information entered into the source records was very limited. Several other subjects were recruited to the study who did not meet the inclusion criteria stated in the protocol and there were several discrepancies in baseline data. The following discrepancies were noted for the selection criteria:

12 subjects: No X-ray – primary diagnosis not confirmed.

11 subjects: According to X-ray, primary diagnosis not confirmed.

8 subjects: Source documents indicated other conditions prohibited by protocol – protocol violations.

5 subjects: The baseline VAS score was below 5 cm – protocol violations.

2 subjects: Subject's X-ray performed more than six months before study–protocol violations.

The medical history as noted in the source medical records had not been adequately described in the CRF for 25 patients. Information recorded in CRFs not recorded or not consistent with information recorded in the source documents. Discrepancies in the use of concomitant medication were noted in a comparison of the source medical records and the CRFs in 30 patients. Not all medication taken in the last three months prior to the study and during the study (required to be recorded according to the protocol), as indicated on the investigators' computerized database, had been entered in the CRF. Discrepancies in AE reporting were noted in a comparison of the source medical records and the CRFs in more than 10 patients.

The main effectiveness variables (pain rating) were recorded in the CRF and the diary cards. Apart from a general statement on efficacy on some stickers and 'summary documents', there were no details in the source medical records to verify efficacy data. It appeared that nurses (not site physicians) were responsible for instructing the subjects on application of the study medication and completion of the diary cards for assessment of pain. The names of more than 10 different nurses were provided to the auditors. There was no evidence of a pre-study meeting to standardise procedures for the nurses and no assessment of inter-rater reliability. There was no evidence that the same nurse was responsible for both pre-study and post-study assessments for the same subjects. In some cases, information in source records indicated 'inefficacy', although the VAS scores indicated improvement. In the CRFs, some original notations on pain scales had been changed and dated by nurses. There was no explanation for why changes were made.

With respect to the VAS, the auditors noted that for several subjects, crosses were used to mark the VAS score, which either did not cross the VAS line at all or crossed it twice. Apparently, the investigators were not instructed to ask the subjects to use a single straight line (and not a cross) perpendicular to the VAS line to mark their score. For some subjects, the lines used to mark the VAS scores were not drawn perpendicular to the VAS line, but oblique. The VAS rating scales in the CRF and the diary cards were required to be completed by study subjects, but for more than 15 subjects, these were modified by study site personnel (usually study nurses). For example, pain at rest was modified from a value < 5 cm (patient ineligible) to a value > 5 cm (patient eligible). Changes were dated and initialled, but no reasons for changes were provided and/or the reason for the change was written as 'crossed in error', or 'misunderstood question'.

CRFs were not all signed and dated by the physicians who were responsible for the study subjects. One signatory who apparently did not see any subjects personally had signed at least 50% of the CRFs. None of the other physicians who were directly responsible for the care of the subjects had signed the

CRFs (with one exception). It was not obvious in the CRO records that subjects were actually seen by the physicians who had signed the CRFs. The auditors questioned the basis on which these individuals had signed as being responsible for the data for subjects they had not personally seen.

CHAPTER 6

Managing Study Medications / Devices

The mismanagement of study medications/devices could result in failure of many studies in our experience. This is a complicated area and yet many clinical researchers report that they are not particularly interested in this aspect of clinical studies and assume that it is all handled by personnel in the manufacturing facility. On the other hand, personnel in the manufacturing facility report that once the supplies are released, they assume no further responsibility! The result is that no one may be ensuring the safety of the product being studied.

While monitors and study site personnel are not normally involved in the direct manufacture of study medications or devices, they should all be concerned about the procedures for requisition, labelling and packaging, before any study subjects are treated, to ensure that a safe product will be issued for clinical studies (section 6.1).

At the time of release of study supplies for shipment from the sponsor/manufacturer to the study sites, there is a dramatic lessening in the level of control of those supplies. Thus all aspects of shipment must be carefully assessed and documented. The documentation of receipt at the study site is also critical (section 6.2).

Evidence of careful control at the study site is imperative and naturally it is difficult to standardise the situation across many study sites and many countries. Security, correct storage, and accurate documentation of dispensing and inventory are critical. Systems to ensure and assess compliance with the required use of the product being studied must be established. Monitors must be trained to check on these features and ensure that all site personnel are fully briefed (section 6.3).

Overall accountability is critical. A reconciliation of the initial inventory and the final returns must be undertaken and all discrepancies must be explained. Final disposition and destruction must be carefully documented to also allow assessment of possible detrimental environmental impact. Accountability may be affected by issues such as recall of products, reallocation of products and use of products outside the approved indication (section 6.4).

Clinical studies usually involve randomisation and blinding procedures to minimise possible bias in assessing results. These procedures are unique to studies of investigational products and yet there is little guidance in guidelines and regulations. Thus, the sponsor/CRO must have a set of carefully developed written procedures and must ensure that site personnel also understand the rules (section 6.5).

Finally, we have also included in this chapter some comments about the procedures for handling, shipping, and collecting biological samples. These procedures must be described for both sponsor/CRO and site personnel to ensure that accurate data are obtained, to ensure that handlers are exposed to the lowest possible risk of contamination with potentially infectious material, and to ensure full accountability of all samples (section 6.6).

6.1 PREPARATION OF STUDY MEDICATIONS/ DEVICES

The preparation of study medications or devices for clinical studies is a time-consuming process and possibly one of the most rate-limiting steps in initiating the study, particularly with double-blind designs.

At the sponsor/CRO site, requisition of study medication/ device (including placebo and comparator products, if relevant) must be initiated at the time of the internal agreement to conduct the study, which may be prior to issue of the final protocol. This is necessary to allow sufficient time to procure the study medication/device and to prepare the final labelling and packaging, taking into account any special circumstances for blind studies and for import requirements.

Requisition of study medications/devices for blind studies requires special consideration: the test medications/devices, active standard controls, and placebos used in a blind randomised study should be indistinguishable by appearance, taste, smell and other physical characteristics; if changes are to be made to any formulation to preserve blindness, then it may be necessary to conduct appropriate bioavailability studies; and a sealed copy of the randomisation code must accompany the request form sent to the packaging organisation.

Also, requisition of study medications/devices from other countries requires special consideration. If it is necessary to import supplies (bulk or packaged) from other countries, then it will be necessary to document inspection of the foreign manufacturing facility and a statement of GMP compliance of the foreign facility must be available in the clinical study file. It will be necessary to determine the rules for import licences. Obtaining marketed products from other manufacturers may necessitate preparation for special purchase orders.

Study medications/devices may be sent from the manufacturing facility to a contract packaging organisation for further distribution to affiliates of a CRO and/or directly to the investigational sites. Before release of investigational products to investigational sites, the following documents must be available in the clinical study file: a GMP statement declaring that suitable standards were met during manufacture and issued by an independent qualified person (e.g. 'Qualified Person' in Europe) who is responsible for approving all components, test article product containers, closures of containers, in-process materials, packaging material, and labelling of study materials, including those prepared by other manufacturers; certificates of analysis, signed and dated for each study medication/device, and clearly indicating the constituents of the batch, the batch number, the expiry date, and any necessary storage requirements; and evidence of retention of samples from each batch. At 90% of 226 study sites in our audit database, there was no evidence, in the clinical study files, of compliance with GMP or retention of samples from batches. These documents were possibly elsewhere, but would anyone else be able to find them in the future?

... A study of stroke, Portugal, 500 patients
This study involved an approved drug in a new indication. The formulation and dose of the study medication differed from the approved product licence – this was not explained in the protocol. Obviously, this situation will raise questions about the comparability of the formulations of the marketed product and the investigational product.

... A study of hormone replacement therapy, Canada, 12 study subjects
Study medication was not prepared at the time study subjects were screened and provided consent. Study subjects should never be recruited into studies in these situations. What would happen if it was eventually determined that the study medication could not be prepared after all? Perhaps the subject had undertaken risky screening procedures for no reason.

The principles of safe labelling and packaging are to ensure that the contents of the container can be identified, that a contact name, address and telephone number is available for emergencies and enquiries, and that the study subject (or the person administering the medication/device) knows how to store and administer the study medication/device. The rules for labelling vary from country to country and this tends to be a complicated area. However, there must be evidence in the clinical study file of compliance with the specific country rules. Checklist 6.1–1 may provide some guidance for labelling, but the reader should seek expert advice. Study site personnel should check that labels provide accurate and clear information to study subjects.

... A study of condition X, several sites in Europe
The study medications were prepared in blister packs with no labelling whatsoever on the packs. The three-treatment arm study was thus

completely blind! Apparently some countries had refused to import the study medication and some study nurses had refused to use the medication because of the labelling. The company carried on with the study anyway and eventually obtained authorisation to market the drug in the UK.

... A study of an antibiotic, Canada, 42 patients
The labels on the study medication containers indicated that 400 mg capsules were being studied: the protocol referred to 500 mg capsules.

The packaging specifications must be reviewed to ensure compliance with the protocol and to ensure that the following requirements are met: suitable types of containers (e.g. cartons, jiffy bags) and grouping of packaging are used; suitable types of packaging (e.g. blister packs, encapsulation) are used; study medications/devices are in childproof containers; and packaging materials are suitable to ensure proper environmental conditions are met. Site personnel should check all labelling upon receipt of investigational supplies. The sponsor/CRO must ensure that study site personnel do not relabel and repackage study materials and the monitor should determine the normal procedures at each clinical site. If the clinical site insists on this practice, the monitor (or perhaps more qualified sponsor/CRO personnel) should witness and document all labelling.

Checklist 6.1–1. General Labelling Requirements

The following items should be included on the primary container labels of study medications/devices:
- Identification, strength and dosage form of the study medication/device (with due attention to the need to maintain blinding, if applicable);
- Quantity of medication in the container. The label must indicate the specific number of capsules, tablets, millilitres, etc. It is not acceptable to write phrases such as 'Supplies for Visit 2'.
- Study identification (e.g. code/number) and abbreviated study title (e.g. 'Osteoporosis Study of X versus Placebo');
- Unique subject identification code (e.g. study subject number, randomisation number, site identification (if multicentre study));

- Instructions for administration, including route of administration and dosage regimen, and instructions for storage/handling. (If vials or ampoules are used for IV administration, it may only be necessary to put this information on the outer packages.)
- A statement that the medication/device is 'For clinical study purposes only';
- Batch number (or 'study code number' for blind studies);
- Expiry date (or 'use before' date for blind studies) or 'retest' date;
- Warnings concerning safety of children, requirements to keep the medication/device at a specific temperature (e.g. refrigerated, frozen, 2 to 8 °C), out of the light, etc. (if relevant);
- Name and address of study site and 24-hour emergency contact telephone number (if not supplied on the emergency contact card provided to the study subject);
- Name/address of manufacturer. Sufficient information must be provided so that the individual using the medication/device can contact someone in the event of emergencies. Local identification, which must be applicable to the country in which the study is being conducted, should be provided.

6.2   SHIPMENT OF STUDY MEDICATIONS/DEVICES

Clinical study medications/devices should not be dispatched to study sites until all pre-study activities have been completed and regulatory requirements satisfied, as described in Chapter 2. A formal authorisation (in the sponsor/CRO records) for the release of clinical study supplies to the study site must be issued prior to any shipment. Special rules for exporting to other countries may require intervention of a local shipping agent or local manufacturing facility. There will also be special rules for controlled substances and quarantine periods may be required for some substances.

Study medication/device shipments must always be accompanied by the shipment letter, a card for the pharmacist/investigator to acknowledge receipt, randomisation codebreak envelopes, if applicable, dispensing forms, inventory forms, forms to document destruction (if permitted at the study site), certificates of analysis, certificates of release, a statement of GMP compliance and a statement of retention of samples. The shipment letter must contain all necessary details about the shipment. In our database, the shipment letter was missing important information at 85% of 378 audited sites. Specific missing information included handling instructions (80%), storage instructions (76%), expiry or use before dates (65%), specific quantity per package (59%), number of packages (51%), method of shipment (50%), shipment date (28%) and specific subject numbers shipped (26%).

The monitor must be notified of all shipments, so that a pre-shipment notification can be sent by the monitor to alert the site (or the affiliate or the CRO, if applicable) that the shipment can be expected. (It is preferable to ship supplies to pharmacies in all clinical settings where pharmacies exist because these facilities have expertise in handling supplies.) The recipient should be instructed to notify the monitor immediately if the shipment does not arrive within a specified time period. The monitor should also confirm receipt by telephone. If, for logistical reasons, it is necessary for supplies to arrive before the initiation visit by the monitor, the site must be instructed to retain the supplies securely under the correct conditions until the monitor arrives at the initiation visit. (It is not likely that the arrival of the supplies will coincide with the initiation visit, unless supplies are hand-carried by the monitor.) If study medications/devices must be stored at the sponsor/CRO premises, prior to shipment to investigators, the storage facilities must also be adequate on those premises.

When supplies are hand-carried by monitors, the procedure must be carefully documented. Security and appropriate environmental conditions must be maintained at all times. (For example, storage in the monitor's vehicle may be inappropriate if extremes of temperature are anticipated.) The monitor should, in general, remain with the study medication/device at all times for security reasons. If special couriers are used, the monitor must ensure that all documents (e.g. shipping invoice, courier, flight details, way bills) are maintained. Provisions must be made to ensure that proper environmental conditions will be maintained at all times during the shipment period. If the assigned carrier cannot meet these requirements, the shipper must institute other measures (e.g. temperature markers in the packaging).

If it is necessary to replace expired supplies during the study, all the above principles must be satisfied. In addition, the following requirements must be considered: provision of authorised stability data to support an extension of the expiry date; certificates of reanalysis; documentation of procedures for requesting subjects to return expired materials and procedures for replacement; provision of updated labels with instructions for relabelling; and necessity for quarantine for returned expired material.

The receipt of each shipment of study medication/device will be confirmed in writing by the investigator or pharmacist (or other authorised personnel) who will be instructed to return a completed 'acknowledgement of receipt form' immediately by facsimile or by use of a self-addressed return envelope, retaining a copy for the study site files. The recipient at the study site will be instructed to telephone the sponsor/CRO immediately if there are any problems (e.g. missing or broken items, defects in labelling, evidence of excursion from temperature ranges) with the shipment. The recipient must be particularly instructed to record the exact date of receipt of the clinical supplies at the study site. (If the form is only signed and dated on the date that it is completed, it may not indicate exactly when the supplies were received.) This information is necessary so that the monitor can determine that the supplies were secure and correctly stored environmentally during the entire period of shipment. The investigator will also be instructed to complete the inventory form (Checklist 6.3–1) immediately.

... A study of hormone replacement therapy, UK, 35 study subjects
A shipment sent on 2 October was apparently received on 6 September in the same year. This fairly common event probably occurs because of sloppy paperwork. Nevertheless, it initially arouses suspicion about the use of the study medication/device.

... A study of dyspepsia, UK, 57 patients
The study medication was apparently received after the first patient entered the study, according to the documentation. Further, several subjects were administered a drug for compassionate use after completion of the study and the new labelling specified the medication container contents. Thus, the double-blinding of the study was probably ruined.

... A study of hormone replacement therapy, UK, 29 study subjects
Study medication shipped on 24 August was acknowledged as received
on 1 November in the same year. There was no explanation for the long
interval or of the conditions maintained during that interval. This
very common occurrence is of great concern since there is basically no evidence that the supplies were maintained securely
and in an intact condition. *The labelling stated 'do not use beyond*
trial period' with no other indication of an expiry date. This does not
provide adequate information at all: would all study subjects
understand the duration of the trial period? *On the sponsor*
premises, the drugs were maintained in a large warehouse which had
no environmental control, no separate storage area for investigational
drugs, no controlled access and no inventory control.

... A study of hormone replacement therapy, Canada, 25 study
subjects
The medication receipt form was signed before medications were
actually received at the study site!

After the clinical study supplies have been sent to the study
site, the monitor must verify as soon as possible that the
supplies have arrived satisfactorily. Safe arrival may be initially
confirmed by telephone and then followed up at the initiation
visit (or at the next monitoring visit if additional supplies are
sent after commencement of the study). The monitor will
verify and document that during the shipment period (defined
as the period from the time of release to the time of acknowledgement of receipt), all conditions for security and correct
storage were maintained. Supplies may not be dispensed to
study subjects until the monitor has checked their condition,
normally at the initiation visit. The monitor will verify that the
amount shipped matches the amount acknowledged as
received. If there is a lack of reconciliation, or if the shipment
is not intact, recruitment may be delayed until the situation is
resolved.

At the initiation visit and prior to any treatment of study
subjects, the monitor will brief the investigator, the pharmacist,
and other concerned site personnel, about the handling and
control of clinical study supplies, and will explain the use of all
forms to document study medication/device use.

6.3   CONTROL OF STUDY MEDICATIONS/DEVICES AT STUDY SITES

Upon receipt of study medications/devices, the study site should initiate and maintain an inventory documenting all receipt and returns (Checklist 6.3–1). (Details required in the inventory might be incorporated into a dispensing list.) The monitor must ensure that the investigator (or pharmacist) also maintains details of dispensed medications/devices for each individual study subject on the dispensing record (Checklist 6.3–2). The monitor will check the medication/device inventory and the dispensing records at each monitoring visit, ensuring that all entries are signed and dated by the investigator or the pharmacist, and the monitor will compare these documents with each other and with other evidence in the CRFs, the diary cards, the shipment forms and the acknowledgement of receipt forms. The monitor will also count and measure supplies, record findings, and report discrepancies. The purpose of these activities is to facilitate the process of reconciliation of all supplies. In our audit database, a study medication/device dispensing list was not maintained at the study site at 26% of 378 sites and the dispensing list was missing important information at 49% of the sites. Specific missing information included: quantity (used or unused) returned to sponsor/CRO (52%); dose prescribed (51%); identification of dispenser (44%); date returned by study subject to pharmacy or study site (42%); name of medication/device (38%); container number (34%); visit number (34%); quantity dispensed (30%); study identification (26%); and date dispensed (24%).

The expectations with regard to maintenance of study medications/devices at study sites focus on security and appropriate environmental conditions. Concerns for security require that supplies be maintained under locked conditions. All agreements between the sponsor/CRO and the study site must specify that supplies are only for clinical study subjects – this information must also be clearly stated on the labelling. The main concern for appropriate environmental conditions is usually temperature requirements, but other factors (e.g. light, humidity) might also be important. Terms such as 'room temperature' and 'ambient temperature', terms which have different meanings in different countries, should always be avoided and specific temperatures must be stated. At each monitoring visit, the monitor will ensure that the correct procedures are being followed. According to our audit database, study medications/devices were not stored safely at the study site (or there was inadequate evidence of safe storage) at 49% of 378 sites. The temperature at which study medication was stored was of particular concern. In some cases, the presence of means of measuring and controlling temperature was absent in environments in which temperatures in excess of 30 °C were likely.

... A study of cardiovascular surgery, UK, six patients
The study medications were retained at the study site in an unlocked domestic refrigerator, with no temperature control. The same refrigerator was used to store milk and food!

... A study with an anxiolytic, UK, 12 study subjects
The study drug was required to be stored at 2–8 °C. On the day of the audit, the temperature in the refrigerator (observed on a thermometer in the refrigerator) was observed as 15 °C. The auditors were informed that this was because they had just opened the door to the refrigerator! One of the auditors almost burned his hand on the autoclave which was adjacent to the refrigerator. The site was also proud of the fact that it maintained daily temperature records: the temperature exceeded the required temperature range every day!

... A study of back pain, UK, 25 patients
The investigator reported that some of the missing drug supplies were in his personal care at home for 'emergencies'. The sponsor had no record of shipment. The drug supply storage area was in the attic of the surgery. The boilers were also in this room – and it was very hot on the day of the audit.

... A study of hormone replacement therapy, France, 15 study subjects
The study medication, required to be stored at 'room temperature', was stored in a room with a steriliser. The auditors conducted the audit in the same storage room and found the room to be very hot.

... A study of hormone replacement therapy, The Netherlands, 21
study subjects
There were several problems with drug supplies which ruined this
study: the investigator was sent supplies from a new randomisation
block although he had not used all medication from the blocks which
had been assigned to him; a drug which was delivered in February
was apparently received in June and there was no explanation for the
long time interval; and randomisation envelopes had been prepared
although the study was not blind! Further, there were numerous
discrepancies between diary cards completed by patients, CRFs and
data printouts. When the auditor could not find an explanation for
the discrepancies in other documentation, she asked to see the physical
evidence (the supplies) in order to conduct a count. The auditor was
informed that returned medication had been destroyed (although the
study was ongoing) because there was not enough room for storage.
Companies should ensure that returned supplies are retained
until after the clinical report is prepared. The cost of storage
space is small compared to the cost of losing a study because
discrepancies cannot be explained.

Compliance with medication/device use (by the study
subject) should be assessed in all studies. In studies in which
supplies are dispensed to subjects for self-administration,
methods to ensure compliance (e.g. diary cards, instructions on
labelling, supervised administration) and methods to check
compliance (e.g. tablet counts, plasma/urine assays, diary card
review) must be in place. At each study visit, the study subjects
should be asked to return all unused supplies and empty
containers to the investigator who will check the supplies for
assessment of compliance and store them for return to the
sponsor/CRO. The monitor will review all relevant documents
(e.g. source documents, CRFs, medication/device inventory,
dispensing forms) to ensure that the data in the CRFs reflect the
subjects' compliance with the study medications/devices.
Details concerning compliance should be entered into the CRF.

... A study of antifungal prophylaxis, UK, 29 patients
The protocol required blood levels of the study medication to be assayed
as a means of determining compliance with use of the study medica-
tion. This was not done.

Our audit database showed that there was inadequate evidence in the monitoring visit reports to indicate that the monitor routinely checked all aspects of management of study medication/ device (e.g. storage, expiry dates, quantity, dispensing, compliance, returns, etc.) at 57% of 378 sites. If the monitor does not regularly and systematically assess the situation, it can only further deteriorate.

Checklist 6.3–1. Study Medications/Devices Inventory

The following items should be specified in an inventory of study medications/devices at each study site:
- Quantity received. (Specify total quantity and amount by study subject.)
- Date received;
- Number of individual study subject package units;
- Study subject numbers of individual study subject package units;
- Treatment period (e.g. visit number);
- Quantity dispensed;
- Quantity returned;
- Quantity unused;
- Quantity destroyed;
- Quantity damaged;
- Balance;
- Explanation for discrepancies.

Checklist 6.3–2. Study Medications/Devices Dispensing Records

The following items should be specified in dispensing records:
- Study subject confidential identifiers;
- Visit number;
- Unit description (e.g. one bottle of 50 capsules);
- Quantity of units dispensed;
- Container number(s);
- Date and time dispensed;
- Method of dispensing (e.g. direct to the study subject, to the ward, etc.);
- Quantity of units returned to pharmacy/study site office;

- Date and time of return to study site;
- Date of return to sponsor/CRO;
- Balance (total and per study subject);
- Confirmation of use according to the protocol;
- Comment on any non-compliance;
- Date of verification (and identification of person conducting verification).

6.4   OVERALL ACCOUNTABILITY OF STUDY MEDICATIONS/DEVICES

An inventory of supplies for the study must be maintained by the sponsor/CRO in addition to the site inventory. In the case of multicentre studies, a complete list of the study sites and supplies dispatched to each site should be maintained. The monitor will check these at each monitoring visit as well as all other documents noted in the previous section. The monitor must also document a summary of medication/device accountability findings on the study closure visit report form (Chapter 7). In our audit database, there were significant discrepancies in the accountability of study medications/devices at 33% of 378 sites. Poor monitoring standards undoubtedly contributed to this finding.

... A study of radio-imaging, Germany, eight patients
On the day of the audit, there was no study medication at the study site. The study was ongoing and some patients were in the middle of a treatment period. Clearly it is unethical to enrol patients in a study unless adequate treatment is available.

... A study of alcohol dependence, Germany, 26 patients
The study involved double-blind treatment followed by open-label treatment. The first patient reached the date for an open-label portion of study when no medications were available. The site continued to treat him in the double-blind phase of the study. How would the data for this patient be interpreted?

... A study of cardiovascular surgery, Germany, 33 patients
The drug inventory was completed by the monitor. This occurs at

many study sites: the researchers forget that dispensing records and inventories are source documents which must not be completed by sponsor/CRO personnel.

All unused and returned medications/devices, empty containers, devices, equipment, etc. which are returned to the investigator by the study subjects, must be stored securely and under correct environmental conditions at the study site until retrieval by the monitor. The monitor will check the supplies returned and verify that they reconcile with the written specifications. All discrepancies and the reasons for any non-returns must be documented and explained. This documentation will be signed by the investigator or pharmacist for each study medication/ device. If the monitor is not hand-carrying returned articles, the study site must be provided with instructions for packaging and shipment. For the return of hazardous and controlled medications/devices, specific guidance will be issued. Local rules for shipment between countries must also be considered.

... A study of hormone replacement therapy, France, 35 patients
The auditors observed an invoice for 200 vials to be sent to the study site. There was no documentation of dispatch or receipt. Several other vials were discarded apparently due to an 'error in manipulation' and several vials were reported as destroyed, but there was no documentation. Several of the alterations in the records were done with white liquid paper to overwrite original entries. It is likely that inspectors would lose confidence in the validity of the study when these kinds of errors all occur in the same study.

... A study of a skin disorder, Germany, 11 subjects
Half of the shipment to the study site (50 of 100 tubes) were not accountable in the dispensing records.

Generally, destruction of returned study medications/devices by the sponsor/CRO may not take place until the final report has been prepared and until there is no further reason to question the accountability of the study medication/device. Authorisation by the sponsor/CRO is necessary and must be documented. Further, the actual destruction process must be documented in a manner which clearly details the final disposition of the unused medications/devices and the method of destruction. The information is particularly necessary in case of any query regarding environmental impact. In exceptional circumstances, unused study medications (e.g. cytotoxics, radio-labelled products) may be destroyed at the study site after written authorisation from the sponsor/CRO has been obtained. For study site destruction, the following considerations must be addressed: no medications should be destroyed at the study until they have been checked by the monitor; the name and credentials of the persons undertaking destruction must be obtained; the destruction facilities must be inspected by the sponsor/CRO; and the site must provide certification that supplies were destroyed in accordance with the sponsor/CRO instructions. Our audit database indicated that the following information was not documented in 226 study sites: method of destruction (96%); date of destruction (89%); quantity broken/unstable (80%); quantity destroyed (80%); discrepancies recorded and explained (55%); date received by sponsor/CRO (49%); and quantity returned (48%).

Most companies adhere to the policy that study medications/devices may not be reallocated from one study site to another. However, if there is no other alternative or if the costs of preparing new supplies are prohibitive, strict rules for reallocation must be followed and must be authorised by the sponsor/CRO. For example, study medications/devices should not be reallocated directly from one study site to another study site, but must first be returned to the manufacturer.

... A study of prostate cancer, UK, 32 patients
The study medication was reallocated from one study site to another. This was undertaken by site personnel and not checked by the company. Pharmacy personnel at the new site repackaged and relabelled all containers and the new labels included the names of the patients. This situation exactly exemplifies the risk of uncontrolled reallocation procedures. Was the repackaging conducted properly given that the study was double-blind? *An open copy of the randomisation code was maintained in the study site files.*

Recall of study medications/devices, requested by the sponsor/CRO, may be necessary because of safety hazards, procedural problems or requests by regulatory authorities. Recall may also be requested when the study is terminated prematurely or abandoned, the study is of long duration and the study supplies are to be replaced at predetermined intervals, or the supplies exceed shelflife. (The exact reason for recall must always be documented.) The clinical safety of subjects is uppermost and determines the method of recall. It may be necessary to wean some subjects gradually off treatment, depending on the characteristics of the study medication/device and some subjects must be immediately discontinued from the study while others may continue until a replacement is provided. All relevant requirements must be documented (e.g. whether recall must be immediate for emergency reasons or is due to normal circumstances such as passing the expiry date). If replacements are to occur, description of the specific procedures for recall and replacement, the identification of all supplies recalled and all replacements, if any, and the placement of recalled products in quarantine, must be documented.

Use of study medications/devices outside the limitations of an approved protocol (e.g. 'compassionate use', 'compassionate plea use', 'unlabelled request use', 'emergency procedure', 'named-patient treatment or supply' and use under a 'treatment IND') is an exceptional procedure and requires authorisation by the sponsor/CRO. It is a procedure to be avoided because of the risk of less rigorous control of the study and the possibility of confounding results and spurious publications. (If the sponsor/ CRO provides an investigational product to an investigator or supports the study of an investigational product (financially or otherwise such as providing support personnel or guidance), the sponsor/CRO is responsible for accountability of the medications or devices and reporting of all safety data. Unapproved use must be prohibited by the sponsor/CRO if: there is insufficient evidence of effectiveness in current clinical studies; a development decision has not been reached; the medication/device is marketed for other indications; the medication/device can be purchased from the country where the medication/device is marketed; and similar medications/devices are available on the market. Conduct of normal clinical studies is always the preferred development strategy of the sponsor/CRO. Usually, the prerequisites for 'emergency' or 'compassionate plea' use include the following: the patient for whom the medication/ device has been requested has been medically judged to be in a life-threatening situation or severely ill; there is evidence that the investigational medication/device is the valid choice in the disease condition; and there is a lack of similarly effective and/or tolerated alternative treatment.

The term 'investigator (doctor/dentist) – initiated' investigations applies to studies in which there is no form of support from the sponsor/CRO. Regulatory authority permission is normally necessary and requires the agreement of the sponsor/CRO. The situation in which investigators wish to continue treatment with an investigational medication/device in patients who have completed a formal clinical study should be avoided. However, if this procedure is permitted, and if it does not involve unblinding the study, a follow-up protocol and CRF, or a protocol amendment, must be considered. In those circumstances where the use of the study medication/device is likely to be for a particular unapproved indication by a large number of 'investigators', an 'unapproved use' protocol and CRF should be prepared to ensure the safe use of the medication/device and the collection of appropriate effectiveness and safety data.

'Investigators' involved in the use of study medications/device outside approved limits will not receive financial assistance and must agree not to publish any clinical observations without providing the opportunity for review by the sponsor/CRO. (Provision of free drug supplies implies support and may be contrary to regulatory requirements.) If the study medications/devices provided for use outside approved limits were not actually used, they must be returned and may not be used for any other study subjects. Any safety information collected from 'unapproved' use must be included in safety updates. Further, the following items must be filed by the sponsor/CRO project archives for all use of study medications/devices outside approved limits: all telephone reports and correspondence; signed and dated letter of agreement; name of 'investigator' and address and institution where patient was treated; copies of communications and/or approval received from health authorities and ethics committees; completed 'CRFs' and copy of 'protocol'; precise description of the medication/device sent to the 'investigator'; outcome (e.g. final disposition) of any unused medication/device; and copies of any publications or abstracts.

Checklist 6.4–1. Items to Consider for Re-allocation of Study Medications/Devices

For re-allocation of study medications/devices, the following items must be confirmed:

- Study medication/device has not been previously dispensed to a study subject;
- Items were originally shipped to the site in packaging which would reveal any tampering;
- No tampering was evident;
- Original shipment of the study medications/devices to the study site was received in good condition;
- Evidence that the medications/devices were stored under the appropriate environmental conditions (as specified in the protocol, the investigator brochure and the labels) both during shipment to the study site and at the study site. The evidence must be in writing and include temperature recording lists from the storage area with confirmation of security.
- Shipment of returned study medications/devices to the sponsor/ CRO was received in good condition;
- Reconciliation of retrieved materials was performed by the sponsor/ CRO and indicated agreement with the original shipment form to the study site, the acknowledgement of receipt forms, and the dispensing records;
- Samples of the re-allocated supplies are retained (if possible) for a re-analysis;
- If site-specific labels were used, these have been removed. All new labelling (e.g. unlabelling, overlabelling, underlabelling) has been authorised;
- The sponsor/CRO regulatory affairs department and the study medications/devices department has been informed of the intended re-allocation and have agreed that returned clinical supplies may be reused.

6.5   RANDOMISATION AND BLINDING

Randomisation procedures are used to ensure that study subjects entered into a comparative study are treated in an unbiased way. Blinding (or masking) procedures (e.g. single-blind or double-blind) further minimise bias by ensuring that outcome judgements are not based on knowledge of the treatment. If the study design is double-blind, it is essential that all personnel who may influence the subject or the conduct of the study, are blinded to the identity of the study medication/ device assigned to the subject and therefore do not have access to randomisation schedules.

When a protocol requiring randomised treatment of patients is available, a randomisation schedule must be requested from the sponsor/CRO's biostatistician who will generate the schedule, ensuring that it meets protocol specifications, including the correct block size. The randomisation schedule must always be provided in a sealed envelope to ensure that no sponsor/CRO personnel directly involved in the management, monitoring or analysis of the study have access to the schedule in the event of an emergency requiring knowledge of an individual study subject's treatment.

... A study of prostate cancer, UK, four patients
An open copy of the randomisation code was in the study files for this double-blind study– it was available to all site personnel. This is not an unusual finding.

Also, for blind studies, individual subject randomisation code-break envelopes will be provided to the investigator and/or the pharmacist at each study site with instructions that the envelopes should only be opened in an emergency. A set of randomisation codebreak envelopes must always be available, on a 24-hour basis. Advice on medical procedures, from qualified sponsor/CRO personnel, must be available. In the event of an emergency, the advice should be available within one hour.

... A study of hormone replacement therapy, UK, 29 study subjects
The randomisation code envelopes contained only the identity of a 'group number'. The group number list was nowhere to be found on the sponsor or investigator premises and thus the emergency envelopes were useless in providing identification of the contents.

Any extension or change to the randomisation schedules or their allocation must be agreed in writing and the biostatistician must be involved in carrying out extensions and changes.

If third-party blinding is necessary (i.e. if it is not possible to ensure the anonymity of the medication/device in a controlled clinical study), the aid of reliable persons in the study centres must be sought before the study begins. He/she must guarantee anonymity and conformance to allocated randomisation treatments and should not be given open randomisation schedules, but only sealed coding envelopes which may only be opened immediately prior to the preparation of the investigational product for application.

The block size should not be revealed to study site personnel, or to the monitor or other clinical research personnel. The biostatistician is responsible for overseeing the distribution for each site and each site should be allocated more than one block. It may be preferable to use random block sizes to further minimise the chance of determining the treatments. Obviously, to preserve the blocking arrangements, study subjects must be treated in the order that they present themselves to the investigator and according to the sequence provided by the randomisation schedule.

During a blind study, randomisation code assignments may only be revealed if treatment of AEs is dependent upon knowledge of the medication/device administered or if the study must be terminated for safety reasons (e.g. SAE, overdose) or if an interim analysis of the data is required by the protocol. Opening of randomisation codebreak envelopes by staff of the sponsor/CRO prior to completion of the study and final data resolution requires written authorization. The only exception is when a medical or other emergency exists and authorization cannot be immediately obtained, in which case other sponsor/CRO employees may have access to the randomisation codebreak envelopes.

If the investigator must open an individual subject randomisation codebreak envelope (e.g. in an emergency) then the procedure provided in the protocol should be followed. When a randomisation codebreak is requested, the emergency physician on duty (at the sponsor/CRO premises) must identify the caller, discuss the situation and provide advice. The caller must be advised to only open the codebreak envelope for the study subject under consideration. After opening, the randomisation codebreak envelope should be resealed, dated and signed by the individual who opened the envelope and implications for further treatment of the study subject must be considered. Any opening of randomisation codebreak envelopes must be fully documented. The monitor must visit the study site immediately after the event to verify that only the appropriate envelope was opened and that the situation was properly documented at the study site.

The randomisation schedule for a blind study will not be revealed to any personnel until all data have been gathered, entered into the computer, clarified, resolved, verified, validated and analysed (i.e. when the database is clean and locked and statistical analysis has been completed on blinded groups). Written authorisation to reveal the randomisation schedule must be obtained.

Following completion of the statistical analysis and after the study has been unblinded, the monitor will collect all randomisation codebreak envelopes from the study site. At the same time, the investigator will be provided with a copy of the randomisation schedule so that he/she can retain a record of treatment allocation for each study subject and record the information in the source documents. (To facilitate this procedure, the monitor might provide coloured labels with treatment identification to place in the source documents.) The returned individual randomisation codebreak envelopes (unopened and opened) must be verified by the monitor.

In our audit database, we have observed significant non-compliance with regard to randomisation procedures. The following events were noted in a sample of 226 sites: provisions were not described in protocols or SOPs to ensure that the investigator was informed of the contents of the randomisation code after it was broken (89%); procedures for revealing randomisation codes in double-blind studies at the end of the study were not described (81%); the CRO did not have emergency randomisation codebreak envelopes (63%); there was no identification of the person/department responsible for randomisation code generation (42%); the sponsor did not have emergency codebreak envelopes (40%); and the sponsor did not have a copy of the randomisation list (29%).

... A study of cardiovascular surgery, Europe, several sites
The study was required to be blinded, but it was difficult to prepare matching formulations. The placebo solution was clear; the active solution was yellow. Thus the solutions were required to be prepared and administered by a third party in the operating theatre. Unfortunately many events spoiled the design of this study: lot numbers and expiry dates were printed on the vials; lot numbers were also noted in the initiation report prepared by the monitor and on the drug dispatch documents in the investigator files; one of the monitor reports indicated that she had checked on supplies (accountability, storage and administration) and thus she would not have been blind to the treatment; at one site, while the auditors were checking the drug supplies in the storage area, the investigator walked in and helped himself to a vial, which clearly identified the treatment; and the labelling indicated that the medication was light-sensitive, but the solutions, after filtration and dilution, were being placed in clear plastic bags! It is not easy to maintain a truly blind study.

... A study of diabetes, Canada, 21 patients
Only the investigator had a copy of the randomisation code: the sponsor could not find a copy.

... A study of cardiovascular surgery, The Netherlands, 15 patients
The study medication was required to be handled by a third party to prevent unblinding of this double-blind study. However, the supplies were sent directly to the investigator (and thus he could observe the contents), not the pharmacy. The monitor reports indicated that he had checked the contents as well: thus the study was not blind to the monitor or the investigator.

... A study of an inhaler for asthma, UK, 10 patients
Three copies of the randomisation list were openly available to the monitor and other staff.

Checklist 6.5–1. Information to Consider in Requests for Randomisation Schedules

The following information must be included in all requests for randomisation schedules:
• Blinding conditions (e.g. single, double, third-party, open);

- Study design (e.g. crossover, parallel, etc.);
- Number of subjects (including required replacement provisions, overage, if any);
- Number of treatments;
- Block size (to be determined by the biostatistician: usually all other clinical research personnel are blind to the block size);
- Stratification groups, if relevant;
- Number of study centres;
- Number of copies of randomisation schedule required and rationale for distribution;
- Requirement for individual randomisation codebreak envelopes, if relevant;
- Labelling of randomisation codebreak envelopes (including emergency contact names and telephone numbers);
- For multicentre studies, the following information is necessary:
  - Single randomisation schedule or separate randomisation schedules for each centre;
  - Consecutive numbering for all centres or independent numbering at each study centre;
  - Number of subjects per centre.

6.6   MANAGEMENT OF CLINICAL LABORATORY SAMPLES

Before collection of any biological samples from study subjects, the monitor must verify (and document in the site selection report and initiation reports) that the study site personnel fully understand the items noted in Checklist 6.6–1.

If sample collection kits are to be provided to the study site by the sponsor/CRO or a contracted clinical laboratory, the following items must be considered: inclusion of appropriate items (e.g. courier documents and bags, padded envelopes, plastic sample containers, special containers and gel packs for deep-frozen transport, proforma invoice papers, rack for tubes, labels, needle holders, needles, sampling tubes, serum tubes, urine containers, storage tubes, carton storage box, pipettes, etc.); the time period necessary between request and shipment of additional or continuation supplies; labelling of tubes (e.g. preprinted or prepared as needed, unique number/

code for each study subject); and expiry dates of items in the kits.

The requirements for completion of the sample analysis request forms (to be included in the collection kits with the collected samples) must be explained by the monitor to study site personnel, addressing all information as noted in Checklist 6.6–2. The request forms should be preprinted with unique numbers and combined use of forms should not be allowed.

Handling of special substances (e.g. radio-labelled substances and unlabelled biological specimens) must be explained by the monitor. Final disposal of any biological samples requires the authorisation by senior sponsor/CRO personnel and must be carefully documented.

... A study of epilepsy, France, 13 patients
One subject was identified as HIV positive. There was no information on the laboratory samples to indicate to personnel the hazardous nature of the samples.

... A study of hormone replacement therapy, Canada, 25 study subjects
During the audit, the auditors observed the study co-ordinator remove several sample collection kits from a domestic freezer and hand them over to a courier. She did not record what she handed over.

Checklist 6.6–1. Study Site Personnel Briefing for Management of Clinical Laboratory Samples

The following items should be discussed with all site personnel with regard to the management of clinical laboratory samples:
- Parameters to be assessed must be in accordance with the protocol;
- Source of sample for each parameter (e.g. serum, plasma, urine, faeces);
- Analysis technique for each parameter;
- Analysis instrument/equipment for each parameter;
- Identification of parameters which might need to be assessed locally (e.g. quick time and partial thromboplastin time and those which will be assessed centrally (if using a central laboratory);
- Procedures for storage, collection (e.g. vacuum sampling, butterfly

sampling system) and shipment (e.g. courier service, hand-carrying by monitor);
- Requirements for fasted samples;
- Requirements and calibration for equipment (e.g. centrifuge).

Checklist 6.6–2. Biological Sample Analysis Request Forms

The following items should be included on request forms for biological sample analysis:
- Study subject identification (only initials and number);
- CRF number;
- Treatment number;
- Sex and date of birth;
- Visit number and date;
- Fasting (if required);
- Time and date of collection (sampling) at study site;
- Time and date of shipment to clinical laboratory;
- Time and date of receipt by clinical laboratory;
- Time and date of analysis of sample;
- Time and date of issue of report to study site;
- Time and date of review of report by investigator;
- Current reference ranges and alert ranges (if applicable);
- Units. (If necessary provide conversion factor if units are different, as well as SI units.)
- Space and instructions for evaluation of each out-of-range parameter;
- Space for indication of problems with sample, if any.

CASE STUDY SIX

A Single-Centre Double-Blind Study of the Pharmacokinetics and Tolerability of Single and Multiple Doses of Drug X in Approximately 30 Healthy Male Volunteers (UK).

This study was conducted at a Phase I facility in the UK (where it is not necessary to seek review or approval from the regulatory authorities for the conduct of Phase I studies). Apart from the serious problems in management of blinding procedures in this study, which basically destroyed the integrity of the study design, many other serious findings were noted by the auditors. This study was the first use of a new investigational drug in humans!

Summary of Major Deficiencies

Standard Operating Procedures: The current SOPs were in the form of one document with a single title page and one document code number. Within this document there were no SOPs on monitoring, closure of a clinical study, or quality assurance. The approval signatures were illegible. A new set of SOPs was apparently to be issued imminently!

Ethics Committee Review: The protocol was reviewed by two committees, a committee set up by the sponsor and an independent committee. The initial single dose phase of the study was approved only by the sponsor committee at the time of screening of study subjects. The single dose phase was approved by the independent committee (by chairperson's action only) on the same day as the first date of dosing: it was not approved at the time of screening of study subjects. For the multi-dose phase of the study, approval was not obtained by any committee until after all subjects had entered the study.

Ethics committee approval by the independent committee was conditional on the inclusion of a specific statement on subject confidentiality, to be added to the information sheet or consent form. There was no evidence that this statement had been added to the forms provided to the study subjects.

A membership list for the independent committee was not available. For the company committee, it was difficult to assess whether or not there was any conflict of interest among the members.

Informed Consent Procedures: The information sheet and consent form lacked clear statements of how subjects' confidentiality would be protected, which was especially important since all subjects were company employees. The inclusion in the consent documents of a specific statement on confidentiality, required and supplied by the independent committee, had not been undertaken.

Protocol: The protocol had been approved by both the company committee (full approval), and the independent ethics committee (chairperson's action), with signatures which predated the final protocol date. Hence, it could not be ascertained which protocol had been submitted to the ethics committees or what had been approved. For both the single-dose and multi-dose phases of the study, subjects had been screened and had received treament before the protocol and a protocol amendment had received full approval from the ethics committees.

The protocol content was deficient in several areas, particularly in the management of AEs, data handling and statistics, and randomisation procedures. The study phase was not clearly specified, but the protocol stated that the study was for the first introduction of the drug to humans. The protocol referred to the occurrence of 'clinically significant' AEs as an endpoint. (This was not further defined.)

The protocol amendment described a different study and should have been issued as a separate protocol. The amendment had not been approved by either ethics committees at the date when subjects were enrolled for the multi-dose phase.

Case Report Form (CRF) Design: The design of the CRF, for the multi-dose phase, was assessed and found to be deficient in several areas. There was no space to record compliance with inclusion and exclusion criteria, or for documentation of previous medications or therapies. There were no instructions to record concomitant medications at each visit. No space was provided to record results of the physical examination, laboratory values and assay results for blood levels of the drug, all of which were required by the protocol.

Setting Up the Study: There was no evidence to show whether the investigator had other clinical research commitments or that he had sufficient time for the protocol. His CV was not present. There was no evidence of a formal assessment of the study site prior to the initiation of the study.

Monitoring: The rate of monitoring was inadequate, and the presentation of monitoring reports was not standardised. Apparently the monitor was not present to observe the initial dosing phases. The monitor reports were deficient in several areas (e.g. recruitment status, protocol compliance, compliance with randomisation procedures, source data verification, management of clinical study supplies and archiving).

Control of Clinical Study Medications: There was no documentation of the method of shipment, handling instructions, storage instructions, study subject numbers, or expiry dates. Study subjects were receiving study medication up to one month after the expiry date recorded on the receipt form. There were no records of return and final disposition of the study medication. Some emergency drug supplies (e.g. isoprenaline and propanalol) were found to be beyond their expiry dates.

The batch and code numbers were present on the study drug labels, which could have led to unblinding of the study by the physician who was dosing the subjects. The protocol required that the drugs be administered by an unblinded physician as there was a potential to distinguish the difference between active and placebo dosing suspensions. (The active formulation was a whitish liquid suspension and the sponsor could not prepare a matching placebo formulation.) The investigator was observed (during the audit) to personally administer the drugs. He assured the auditors that he did not look into the containers as he was administering the drug!

The medications were required to be stored between 2 and 8 °C. The temperature of the refrigerator where the supplies were stored was not routinely monitored and two thermometers inside the refrigerator were non-functional (one had a broken mercury column and one was frozen in an icy coating).

The randomisation code list, held by the nurse at the sponsor site, was open and had never been sealed. The bioanalyst possessed a copy of the randomisation code and routinely analysed blood samples from subjects on active drug in advance of those on placebo. The bioanalyst was also one of the healthy volunteers so he knew what he was receiving!

Filing/Archiving: All study files were maintained at the sponsor site and some important documents were not present in the files. There were no written policies with regard to the required periods for retention of documents. There were no archives at the Phase I facility.

Source Data: There was evidence of notification of the subjects' primary care practitioners, but the notification letters stated that the study had been approved by the ethics committees, which was not the case. (Full approval by the independent ethics committee was obtained after the date of the primary care practitioner letters).

Out-of-range laboratory values were not flagged in the laboratory reports and there was no systematic assessment of these values for clinical significance by the investigator.

Completed CRFs for six of the subjects from the single-dose phase had not been signed by the investigator, although data had been entered several months earlier.

CHAPTER 7

Final Stages in Clinical Studies

At the end of the active clinical research process at study sites, many other issues must be considered for completion of studies. All clinical studies need closure and formal procedures must be followed.

Closure of a study site involves checking that all the documentation is complete, arranging for collection of unused supplies and ensuring that the investigator is aware of any ongoing responsibilities such as the follow-up of subjects and archiving all relevant documentation for the required time period. Closure must be carefully documented. Sometimes, studies must be suspended or terminated prematurely and formal procedures must be followed for these unusual situations (section 7.1).

The final result of the clinical research activity, as far as the clinical research department and the study site is concerned, is normally the clinical report. The 'customer' who will receive this report is the regulatory authority (in the case of pharmaceutical companies who are seeking licensing approval) and obviously the regulatory authority must be sent the best product possible. However, whatever the final objective, all studies must be reported: it is unethical and unscientific to censor data. Therefore, it is important to understand and follow standardised procedures for preparation of final clinical reports (section 7.2). (The next stage, compiling a submission for marketing authorisation, is not dealt with in this book because it is normally under the control of a 'regulatory affairs department' and is worthy of another book!)

Finally, it is critical to appreciate that study documents should be treated as 'precious gold' at both sponsor/CRO and investigator sites. Systems must be in place to ensure that documents will be securely retained for a long period of time (section 7.3).

7.1   CLOSURE OF CLINICAL STUDIES

A study closure visit at each study site is required when all study subjects have completed the last visit and all follow-up activities have been conducted. Prior to the visit, the monitor will review previous monitoring visit reports and correspondence for any outstanding items and will assemble all items which need clarification and take these to the study site for resolution. After the closure visit, the monitor must complete a study closure report. Further guidance on the specific items to be addressed at closure visits is covered in Checklist 7.1–1.

Our audit findings at 226 study sites indicated that many important items were not apparently addressed at study closure: clinical laboratory investigations were not complete and documented (90% of sites); investigators were not reminded to follow up on study subjects (80%); investigators did not have continuing access to randomisation code envelopes (until the treatment allocation was openly revealed) (69%); there was no documentation that any unused medication/device was disposed or destroyed appropriately (60%); investigators were not given instructions to maintain archives for at least 15 years (46%); investigators did not retain secure archives with copies of all required documents (40%); investigators did not retain a list to identify treatment allocation to study subjects (38%); monitors did not complete a study closure report (28%); and monitors did not collect clinical supplies (used containers/ unused supplies) (22%).

Some clinical studies may be required to be prematurely

terminated or suspended. (Suspension refers to temporary discontinuation of the study or a specific study site and the possibility of resumption of the study is implied. Until resumption is effected, the conditions of termination apply, unless there are other provisions in the suspension notice or statement.) Some of the reasons for suspension or termination of studies include: data demonstrating or strongly suggesting that the study treatment (or participation in the study) is unsafe; data demonstrating that the study medication/device lacks sufficient effectiveness to justify continued withholding of effective alternative therapy; protocol or conduct of the study is flawed such that the safety or rights of study subjects may be adversely affected or the validity of the study may be adversely affected; the ethics committee/IRB has withdrawn approval for the study (or is considering new information) and has denied reconsideration; poor recruitment such that it is unlikely that the study will come to completion; relocation of the investigator or reallocation of investigator time or responsibilities, or disqualification of the investigator by order of a regulatory authority; and change of research strategy or change of management priorities. (However, changes cannot be based on a 'whim': any strategy changes must be fully justified as termination of studies can have serious repercussions for study subjects.)

All recommendations for termination or suspension must be supported by a report prepared by assigned sponsor/CRO personnel stating the reasons and the relevant facts. It will be necessary to inform the appropriate regulatory authorities and ethics committees in all cases. If a clinical study must be terminated immediately, the sponsor/CRO must contact the investigator by telephone and issue a follow-up letter on the same day. The sponsor/CRO must also inform the investigator of the procedures to be taken (e.g. continue treatment, titration, substitute alternative therapy, reporting requirements, management of medication/device and completion of CRFs, etc.) for the subjects who are currently enrolled. If the study has been terminated by the investigator, a letter of notification should be sent by the investigator to the sponsor/CRO. The investigator must be reminded of ongoing responsibilities.

Checklist 7.1–1. Procedures at Study Closure Visits

The sponsor/CRO monitor must undertake and document the following procedures at study site closure visits:

- Source data verification completed and documented, all data queries collected, previous protocol violations (if applicable) discussed and discrepancies confirmed, and investigator reminded of continuing role in clarifying data until the database is clean and closed, plans discussed for another visit to review queries (if necessary), follow-up of study subjects documented and investigator reminded of responsibility for further follow-up of study subjects (if required), all SAE documentation collected, and confidential subject identification list complete;
- Medication/device accountability form completed, inventory sheet completed, all unused medications/devices (and empty containers) returned, destruction of medications/devices discussed, randomisation codebreak envelopes all present and collected, randomisation codebreak envelopes left at study site until study unblinded (unmasked) (in this case, arrangements must be made for collection of randomisation codebreak envelopes at a later date), assay samples collected, transport of samples arranged;
- All CRFs (unused and completed) including diary cards and quality of life questionnaires collected, other unused documents (e.g. blank consent forms) and all loaned equipment collected;
- Ethics committee/IRB notified of study completion and plans to notify ethics committee/IRB of final report or summary of study discussed;
- Investigator informed of requirement to sign a copy of the final clinical report (when the clinical study report has been completed, it may be necessary for the monitor to return to the investigator site and obtain his/her signature on the final clinical report), publication policy discussed;
- Study archives complete and secure, arrangements made for missing documents (if any) to be sent to the study site (a follow-up visit may be necessary to confirm that documents have arrived at study site), investigator instructed to retain all documents associated with the study for at least 15 years, retention of records discussed and arranged and agreement to archive documents signed and dated by the investigator;
- Final payments arranged taking into account agreements with regard to reviewing data.

7.2   FINAL CLINICAL REPORTS

Every clinical study undertaken must be described in a clinical study report, whether or not the study is fully completed as planned in the protocol. (In the case of a study that is not fully completed as specified, the format of the report may be a shortened version, stating clearly the reasons why the study was not completed as planned.) Publications, manuscripts, books, and presentations at meetings cannot substitute for formal clinical study reports because the latter must be prepared in accordance with a specified format. Expert guidance is needed for preparation of clinical reports and they are usually written by the sponsor/CRO, rather than the investigator, because of the special requirements.

The clinical study report will be reviewed and approved by the sponsor/CRO before being released to the investigators, ethics committees/IRBs or other external reviewers. Sponsor/CRO authorization should include a medically qualified expert and a biostatistician. Thereafter, the sponsor/CRO-approved clinical study report must be signed by the investigator (in a single-centre study) or by the assigned principal/main co-ordinating investigator in the case of a multicentre study. However, it is a good idea to obtain the signatures of all investigators who make significant contributions to the conclusions of the report. Copies of all signature pages should be retained by both the sponsor/CRO and the investigators, and a list of recipients of clinical study reports should also be maintained by the sponsor/CRO to assist in accountability of these documents.

... A pharmaceutical company requested an audit of five clinical reports which had been submitted to the regulatory authorities as 'model' reports of GCP compliance. The auditors found many errors, particularly with regard to safety data. Also, the data referenced in the statistical report did not always match the data referenced in the clinical report. As a result, the reports had to be withdrawn, which was very embarrassing for the company. This should never happen if there is a good review procedure in the company.

7.3   ARCHIVING

The purpose of archiving is to safeguard all documentation which provides evidence that a clinical study has been conducted in accordance with the principles of GCP. Therefore, archives should be organised so that they are secure but can be easily reviewed by an internal or external auditor. Archives at both the sponsor/CRO and investigator sites must be reasonably secure with regard to indexing, controlled access, fire resistance, flood resistance, etc. In our audit database, a review of 226 investigator sites indicated that files were not reasonably secure at 40–50% of sponsor or CRO or investigator premises. Also, numerous critical documents were missing from archives at these sites, further indicating a lack of control of the documentation.

At the beginning of the study, the sponsor/CRO will initiate their own clinical study archives (Checklist 7.3–1): the monitor will also initiate a secure archiving system at each investigator site (Checklist 7.3–2). (The reader should also refer to the archiving list in the ICH document.) A separate investigator file should be maintained at each study centre in a multicentre study.

Original documents must immediately be directed to sponsor/CRO archives by the monitor as soon as they are retrieved from the study site. The monitor should only keep working copies in his/her files. Original documents, must not be removed from the archives and if information is required from the archives, only photocopies should be provided. Further, original documents should not be sent through the postal system but should be either hand-carried by the monitor or sent by courier. Obviously, all copies submitted to the archives must be legible.

The investigator must be held responsible for ensuring that all source documents, especially records acquired in the normal practice of care and treatment of a study subject, are safely archived and available for inspection by authorised company personnel or regulatory authorities. The monitor, of course, must explain the requirements to site personnel and must check on compliance. If the investigator moves, retires, dies or withdraws from an investigation, the responsibility for maintaining the records must be transferred to a designated individual and the sponsor/CRO must receive notice of the transfer (and agree to the transfer). In some countries, there are specific rules with regard to policies for archiving when patients move or die and the policies must be ascertained at the beginning of the study. If the investigator cannot manage (e.g. organise or finance) suitable storage facilities, the monitor can make arrangements for independent storage. However, the investigator must always have control of off-site storage requirements: the sponsor/CRO should not have access to investigator archives.

The investigator must archive all necessary documents for a minimum of 15 years – the usual industry standard, although this is stated differently in the ICH document. All appropriate clinical study documents should be archived by the sponsor/CRO essentially for the lifetime of the product. The location and security of study site documents and off-site documents must be reviewed on at least an annual basis by the monitor.

Data obtained on magnetic media (floppy diskette, tape), or optical disk, will be archived in the same manner as paper documents. However, electronic data must also be stored away from magnetic fields and excessive heat. Where problems in reading tapes or disks are foreseen, 'hard' (paper) copies must be taken for archiving. In practice, we observe that few companies are willing to destroy paper copies in spite of sophisticated electronic archiving systems.

... A study of diabetes, Canada, 21 patients
The sponsor archives were protected from fire by water sprinklers. All items were in paper format! This is a common occurrence.

... A study of an anticoagulant, Italy, 10 patients
The on-line computer system for randomisation required the investigator to provide the full subject name to the CRO prior to issue of treatment allocation. Full names were maintained on the database of the CRO. To ensure confidentiality, the sponsor/CRO should never retain any documents with study subject names in their archives.

Checklist 7.3–1. Typical Documents in Sponsor/CRO Archives

The following documents will be retained in the sponsor/CRO archives for clinical studies:

- SOPs, SOP review and approval forms, SOP compliance statements, list of recipients, request for SOP waivers, if any, report of SOP violations, if any;
- Sponsor/CRO personnel list, personnel qualifications and experience records, personnel training records, job descriptions, organisation charts;
- Ethics committee/IRB correspondence, review/approval letter, membership list, operating procedures, consent forms/subject information sheet (master copy only, not signed copies);
- Investigator brochure, acknowledgement of receipt, list of recipients;
- Protocol and protocol amendments review and approval forms (internal signatures), signed final protocol and protocol amendments (external signatures), list of recipients, CRF (master copy), CRF review and approval forms;
- Regulatory authority approval/review documents, audit certificates, if any;
- Pre-study assessment visit reports, assessment of CRO, assessment of clinical laboratory, evidence of personnel qualifications, clinical laboratory accreditation and/or certification, laboratory reference ranges, investigator agreements (e.g. responsibilities, finances, confidentiality, insurance/indemnity), site initiation reports, site personnel list; monitoring visits reports, list of monitoring visits, telephone contact reports, correspondence, closure report;
- Completed CRFs, source data verification forms, SAE reports, CRF tracking forms, CRF review forms, data query forms, data query tracking forms, data conventions form, subject classification forms, approved statistical analysis plan, clinical study report review and approval forms, list of recipients, final clinical reports, final statistical report;
- Certificates of analysis, GMP certification, record of batch retention, study medication/device requisition forms, authorisation for release of clinical study supplies, shipment forms, acknowledgement of receipt, inventory forms, dispensing forms, documentation of return, final reconciliation and certificate of destruction forms, randomisation code list and randomisation emergency codebreak envelopes.

Checklist 7.3–2. Typical Documents in Investigator Archives

The following documents will be retained in the study site archives for each clinical study:

- Ethics committee/IRB correspondence, review/approval letter, membership list, operating procedures;
- Investigator brochure, acknowledgement of receipt;
- Signed final protocol and protocol amendments;
- Subject registration form;
- Source documents;
- Completed consent form/information sheets and consent forms/ subject information sheets (master copy);
- Completed CRFs, completed data query forms, CRF (master copy); SAE reports, if any
- Regulatory authority approval/review letter;
- Study site personnel qualifications forms, clinical laboratory accreditation and/or certification, laboratory reference ranges, investigator agreements (e.g. finances, confidentiality, insurance/indemnity agreements), correspondence, records of start up meetings in multi-centre studies, site personnel list (we recommend that copies of initiation reports, monitoring reports and closure reports should also be retained at the study site to help the site personnel and to provide evidence of monitoring activities.);
- Certificates of analysis, GMP certification, shipment forms, acknowledgement of receipt forms, inventory forms, dispensing forms, documentation of return, final reconciliation and certificate of destruction forms, randomisation code list, randomisation emergency codebreak envelopes;
- Clinical study report review and approval forms (external), final clinical study reports;
- Audit certificates, if any.

CASE STUDY SEVEN

Two Multicentre Studies of the Safety and Efficacy of Drug X in Approximately 200 Patients with Disease X (Several Sites World-wide)

The quality of final clinical study reports depends on receiving accurate information and clearly the wrong conclusions may be drawn if the data are not carefully reviewed. Two serious problems were evident in this audit of two clinical study reports. First, there were some serious deficiencies in the reporting of safety data such that the safety profile was probably not adequately represented because of under-reporting. Second, because this audit provided a unique opportunity to review and compare data for the same patients in the two studies – on the same day that some patients completed Study A they were entered into Study B for continuation treatment – we observed that many data with regard to medical history and events, and baseline presentation, were different even in the same patients treated by the same investigators! We reviewed only a small sample of the data.

Summary of Major Findings

Data Errors Relating to Safety: Some examples of discrepancies noted by the auditors in a small audit sample of study subjects included the following:

- A data query form indicated that 'increased diarrhoea' was present at baseline: this was not noted in the data listing. If the event was present at baseline, was it appropriate to be subsequently reported as an AE?
- Under the category 'Other' in the data listing, the entry was 'Yes': this was not in the CRF. The details of the abnormality ('trembling and shaking of arms intermittently') described in the data listing was also not in the CRF. A data query form was issued with the comment 'investigator unco-operative, answered all ? as unknown'. If this was so, where did the information come from?
- The CRF indicated that 'drug X' was prescribed for 'headache' and 'pain in the bladder region'. This was not recorded in the data listing. Was this indicative of new AEs?
- The indication for 'drug X' was recorded as 'prophylaxis' (data listing). A fuller explanation should have been provided: was this indicative of an AE? Only 'antibiotic' was listed for 'perioperative prophylaxis' (data listing). Were no other medications issued during the hospitalisation period, especially during the surgical procedure?

- The indication for 'drug X' was 'abdominal pains' (data listing): this was not reported as an AE.
- The indication for 'infection' should have been more clearly specified (data listing).
- The indication for treatment at visit X was 'pyrexia chest infection' (data listing). 'Pyrexia' was not listed as an AE. The indication 'analgesia' (data listing) should have been more clearly specified.
- The indication for treatment at visit X was 'anxiety-paranoia' (data listing). This event was not listed as an AE.
- The start dates for 'athlete's foot' and 'headache' noted in page x of the data listing was not consistent with any of the dates for AEs noted on page y of the data listing. Were these events indicative of new AEs?
- At the visit X physical examination, 'skeleton/muscles' was listed as abnormal. (It had been noted as normal at baseline.) This was described as 'painful left hip-joint with restricted movements'. Should it have been described as an AE?
- During the study, the subject's weight changed by 10 to 20 kg (data listing). The weight change was apparently not queried. Was it indicative of an AE? (This occurred in at least 5 subjects in the sample.)
- The physical examination at visit X indicated a 'cholecystectomy scar' (data listing). Was a cholecystectomy done during the study? Should an AE have been reported?
- 'Rash groin' was noted as an abnormality at physical examination for visit X (data listing). This was not reported as an AE.
- Was the comment 'mildly sleepy' (data listing) indicative of an AE?
- Were any of the comments for neurological examination (data listing) indicative of AEs? (These events occurred in at least three subjects in the audit sample.)
- Did the comment for visit X indicate that the out-of-range laboratory value was clinically significant? Was this indicative of an AE?
- The pregnancy test was negative at visit X, positive at visit Y, and negative at visit Z. Was the pregnancy normal?
- Several out-of-range values were considered as not clinically significant. As comments were provided for these values (data listing), were they actually clinically significant? Were

they indicative of AEs? (This occurred in at least six subjects in the audit sample.)

- A comment was provided for the abnormal EEG at visit X (data listing). Was this indicative of an AE? (This occurred in at least four subjects in the audit sample.)
- 'Pain in side', listed as the reason for an ultrasound of stomach (data listing), was not recorded as an AE.
- 'Repeated glycemia' was a comment in the data listing. Should this have been reported as an AE?
- The data listing indicated that a 'prescription drug' was associated with the SAE. Since no new entries of concomitant medications were noted during the period of the SAE, the auditors could not determine which drug was prescribed.
- For the event noted at visit X, the data listing indicated that a procedure was undertaken, but the CRF indicated that a procedure was considered but never undertaken. 'Rash scaly' was further described as '... differential fungal rash or drug eruption'. Should the relationship to study drug have been described as 'possible'?
- The AE 'infection' as described in the data listing should have been more specific. The severity for back pains was described as 'unknown' (data listing) but the reported term was 'severe back pains'.
- 'Insomnia' was indicated as not present at baseline (data listing, page x): however, the start date of insomnia on page y of the data listing preceded the start of the study.

Comparison of Data in the Same Patients in Study A and Study B: The following discrepancies were observed by the auditors in a small audit sample:

- The number of doses in the Study B data listing was not consistent with information in the data listing for Study A (10 subjects).
- Some treatments apparently started during Study A (according to the data in the Study B data listing) but were not noted in Study A data listing (nine subjects).
- For medical history and baseline presentation, certain conditions were noted to be abnormal in one listing but not the other listing (e.g. asthma, allergy, depression) (nine subjects).

- Several adverse events were described as 'still present' at the end of the study in Study A data listings, but these items were not observed in the Study B data listings (nine subjects).
- Various treatments were described as 'still present' at the end of the study in Study A listings, but these items were not observed in the Study B data listings (nine subjects).

READING LIST

Australia

Guidelines for Good Clinical Research Practice (GCRP) in Australia, Therapeutic Goods Administration, Commonwealth Department of Health, Housing and Community Services, December 1991.

Canada

Clinical Trial Review and Approval, Drugs Directorate, Policy Issues, Health and Welfare Canada, 1995.

Code of Ethical Conduct for Research Involving Humans, Medical Research Council of Canada, Natural Sciences and Engineering Council of Canada, Social Sciences and Humanities Research Council of Canada, 1998.

European Union

Biostatistical Methodology in Clinical Trials in Applications for Marketing Authorizations for Medicinal Products, Committee for Proprietary Medicinal Products [CPMP] EEC 111/3630/92-EN, 1994.

Clinical Investigation of Medical Devices for Human Subjects, EN540, European Committee for Standardization (CEN), 1993.

Commission Directive 91/507/EEC modifying the Annex to Council Directive 75/318/EEC on the approximation of the laws of Member States relating to the analytical, pharmacotoxicological and clinical standards and protocols in respect of the testing of medicinal products, Official Journal of the European Communities, 1991.

Good Clinical Practice for Trials on Medicinal Products in the European Community, Committee for Proprietary Medicinal Products [CPMP] EEC 111/3976/88-EN, 1990.

Guideline Standard Operating Procedures for Good Statistical Practice in Clinical Research, PSI (Statisticians in the Pharmaceutical Industry), 1993.

Manufacture of investigational medicinal products, *Annex to the EC Guide to Good Manufacturing Practice*, EEC 111/3004/91-EN, 1992.

France

Good Clinical Practices/Bonnes Pratiques Cliniques, Bulletin Officiel de Ministère des Affaires Sociales et de l'Emploi et Ministère Chargé de la Santé et de la Famille, 1987 (English translation).

Protection of Persons Undergoing Biomedical Research/Protection des Personnes qui se Prêtent à des Recherches Biomédicales, Tome 1, Dispositions Législatives, Ministère de la Solidarité, de la Santé et de la Protection Sociale, 1990 (English translation).

Nordic Countries

Good Clinical Trial Practice, Nordic Guidelines, Nordic Council on Medicines, NLN Publication No. 28, 1st edn, December 1989.

Law on a Scientific Committee System and Handling of Biomedical Research Projects, Law No. 503 [Denmark], June 1992.

The Danish Central Scientific Ethical Committee. Collection of Annexes 1994, Den Centrale Videnskabsetiske Komité, 1994.

Spain

Royal Decree 561/1993 of April 16, Establishing the Requisites Concerning Clinical Trials on Drugs, 1993.

UK

Clinical Trial Compensation Guidelines, ABPI, 1994.

Good Clinical (Research) Practice, ABPI, 1992.

Guidelines for Good Pharmacy Practice in Support of Clinical Trials in Hospitals, Royal Pharmaceutical Society, 1994.

Guidelines for Medical Experiments in Non-Patient Human Volunteers, ABPI, May 1990.

Guidelines for Phase IV Clinical Trials, ABPI, 1993.

Guidelines on the Conduct of Investigator Site Audits, ABPI, 1993.

Guidelines on the Practice of Ethics Committees in Medical Research Involving Human Subjects, Royal College of Physicians of London, 1996.

Guidelines on the Structure of a Formal Agreement to Conduct Sponsored Clinical Research, ABPI, 1996.

Local Research Ethics Committees, Department of Health, 1991.

Research Involving Patients, Royal College of Physicians of London, 1990.

Research on Healthy Volunteers, Journal of the Royal College of Physicians of London, **20** (4), 1986.

Standards for Local Research Ethics Committee, Department of Health, 1994.

USA

Code of Federal Regulations, 21 CFR Ch 1: Part 50 – Protection of Human Subjects; Part 56 – Institutional Review Boards; Part 312 – Investigational New Drug Application; and Part 314 – Application for FDA Approval to Market a New Drug or Antibiotic Drug, Food and Drug Administration (FDA), 1998.

Compliance Program Guidance Manual, Chapter 48 – Bioresearch monitoring – human drugs, subject: *in vivo* bioequivalence, FDA, 1990.

Compliance Program Guidance Manual, Chapter 48 – Bioresearch monitoring – human drugs, subject: clinical investigators, FDA, 1994.

Compliance Program Guidance Manual, Chapter 48 – Bioresearch monitoring – human drugs, subject: sponsor/CROs, contract research organizations and monitors, FDA, 1994.

Compliance Program Guidance Manual, Chapter 48 – Bioresearch monitoring – drugs and biologics, subject: institutional review boards, FDA, 1994.

Guideline for the Monitoring of Clinical Investigations, FDA, 1988.

Guideline on the Preparation of Investigational New Drug Products (Human and Animal), Department of Health and Human Services, FDA, April 1991.

Information Sheets for Institutional Review Boards and Clinical Investigators, FDA, Revised October 1995, Reprinted March 1996.

International

Clinical Safety Data Management: Definitions and Standards for Expedited Reporting, International Conference on Harmonisation (ICH) of Technical Requirements for the Registration of Pharmaceuticals for Human Use, 1994.

Declaration of Helsinki. Recommendations Guiding Physicians in Biomedical Research Involving Human Subjects, Adopted by the 18th World Medical Assembly, Helsinki, Finland, June 1964, amended by the 29th World Medical Assembly, Tokyo, Japan, October 1975, the 35th World Medical Assembly, Venice, Italy, October 1983 and the 41st World Medical Assembly, Hong Kong, September 1989, and the 48th General Assembly, Somerset West, Republic of South Africa, October 1996.

Good Clinical Practice: Consolidated Guideline, ICH, 1996.

International Ethical Guidelines for Biomedical Research Involving Human Subjects, Council for International Organizations of Medical Sciences (CIOMS) in collaboration with the World Health Organization (WHO), 1993.

Note for Guidance on Structure and Content of Clinical Study Reports, ICH, 1995.

WHO Guidelines for Good Clinical Practice (GCP) for Trials on Pharmaceutical Products, Division of Drug Management and Policies, World Health Organization, 1994.

Index